REST IS RADICAL
A guide to deep relaxation through yoga

Mel Skinner

D1595944

AEON

First published in 2020 by
Aeon Books
PO Box 76401
London W5 9RG

British Library Cataloguing in Publication Data

Illustrations by Polly Thornhill

A C.I.P. for this book is available from the British Library

ISBN-13: 978-1-91350-418-2

Typeset by Medlar Publishing Solutions Pvt Ltd, India
Printed in Great Britain

www.aeonbooks.co.uk

REST IS RADICAL

To all the teachers I have known, including those
who did not know they were teachers.
Thank you.

CONTENTS

CHAPTER ONE

Welcome

Rest (verb and noun):
cease, abstain, or be relieved from exertion, action, movement, or employment; freedom from or the cessation of exertion, worry, activity, etc.

Radical (adjective and noun):
of the root or roots; far reaching, thorough

Welcome to this book, and welcome to Radical Rest. Learning how to radically rest can help you boost your physical health, develop stronger emotional resilience, and even change the way you perceive yourself and the world around you. This is lying down to wake up, and will help you experience deep relaxation like never before. In this book I will introduce the nine principles and the yoga practices which form Radical Rest, as well as exploring how symptoms of depression, anxiety, addiction, and more can be supported with the practices I share. The principles provide the foundation and guidelines of Radical Rest while the practices give us an embodied way of understanding and exploring the principles through the felt experience of slowing down. This is an invitation to move towards stillness, and in doing so discover a life more peaceful, contented, and joyful.

1

Radical Rest shows us how a more restful approach to life can ultimately create a more fulfilling life. By creating more time and space in your diary to rest in a way which nourishes the body and mind, you could improve your physical, mental, and emotional health and begin to find ways to live your life with greater ease and satisfaction. When we accept and respond to our need to rest in a relentless world, we show a sense of compassion to ourselves and we treat ourselves and our energy with respect. This kindness expands our capacity for understanding not only our own needs to rest, but the needs of our family, colleagues, and even of the environment to regularly rest.

Radical Rest is not about self-improvement (although aspects of your life may improve), but rather an invitation to rest in the person you currently are in order to become the person you could be. As the psychologist Carl Rogers once said, "The curious paradox is that when I accept myself just as I am, then I can change."[1] Radical Rest is a practice of self-acceptance, of seeing our natural flows of energy and enthusiasm alongside our natural ebb towards introspection and quietness, and not favouring one over the other. The more we can find spaciousness in our body, mind, and breath, the more we will find life starts to flow a little more freely for us. Not only that but we will be able to respond to anything tough that life throws at us, rather than falling apart because we are already overwhelmed. We avoid the straw that breaks the camel's back.

Despite the lure of social media and modern advertising to convince us otherwise, we are not designed to be living "our best life" 24/7, but the pressure to be achieving and active at all times is very powerful. We might long for deep and nourishing rest but be unable to give ourselves permission to take it. I felt like this for a long time, and told myself I was happy being busy all the time, even when I was exhausted. In my twenties I even got away with it for a while! Radical Rest really has radically changed my life, but it wasn't always easy to let those changes happen. I congratulate you for picking up this book, because the culture you are most likely embedded in does not advocate doing less: rather you are probably surrounded by billboards of unattainable body images to aspire to, consumerist desires over spiritual wealth, and endless inspirational memes popping up on social media encouraging you to push harder and "resist" tiredness.

Like I once was, perhaps you are burnt out, numb, and disconnected. Perhaps you are ready for another way, but you don't know where to begin. The time to rest really is now, not only for our own health and well-being but for the survival of our soil, endangered species, and the generations to come. It took David Attenborough to draw the attention of the world to the plastic in the sea, but these problems aren't new and while technology may have enabled us to ignore the cycles of the sun and moon, of summer and winter, our Earth has not forgotten that there are times of blossom and plenitude, and times of quiet and dark.

We live in complicated environmental times, and *Rest Is Radical* is my humble contribution towards encouraging you to embody what it is to slow down, pause, cease activity, and rest. If we can experience in our own bodies what nature around us demonstrates each winter (hibernation, dear ones), then we may be able to truly feel how compelling the need to rest really is. When we allow ourselves to step out of busy mode, and instead take deep rest (which incidentally won't cost you a penny, once you know how), then we might also be able to wake up to the idea that we are more than consumers, more than bodies and minds, and more than the beliefs and ideas that we carry. This realisation is a wake-up call that we urgently need, and Radical Rest is one way to slow down the lifestyles and change the systems which are burning out our bodies, and our Earth.

Just before we leap into saving the planet, you may find yourself wondering, *how can **rest** be radical*? Surely this is a contradiction—how could the state of rest possibly bring about any change, least of all something radical? You may even think that resting is unproductive, lazy, pointless or just unnecessary (although if you're reading this I am guessing you already think slightly differently), or you may completely understand why resting would be good for your health but can't understand how it could possibly make any real impact in the world. Pause for a moment. We will come to that, I promise, but pause for a moment. Let the idea roll around on the tongue, *rest is radical*. Does part of you want it to be true? Is there a part of you which longs for deep and nourishing rest which benefits yourself and your world? And now ask yourself:

- When was the last time you were truly relaxed?
- Is rest something you save up for weekends or holidays?
- Have you bought into the idea that resting is something you do when sick, or something only lazy people do?
- When did you last feel really well?

We are told that we are wealthier and healthier than ever before with increasingly advanced technology at our fingertips. When I started researching this book, the hashtag #wellness was featured on over 18 million Instagram posts. In the final edits three years later, that had gone up to almost 30 million and is probably way over that as you read this.[2] Wellness is trending, yet burnout, stress, and exhaustion are no longer terms saved for A-list celebrities and high-powered CEOs, but everyday words bandied around the office and across coffee shop tables as epidemics of tiredness sweep our lands. We are busy and exhausted but we rarely stop. Our diaries are crammed full with appointments, deadlines, and things to do and the notion of "downtime" has become so precious and rare that when we do stop, we can feel depressed, empty, or anxious.

The combination of adrenaline, sugar, and caffeine sets us up in a state of overstimulation which we can confuse as energy. We often associate this feeling with success and vitality, and so when we give ourselves that long-awaited day off, we can feel as though we have crash-landed, feeling worse than we did when we were tired but wired. This is a cycle which tempts us to stay in the overstimulation zone, and results in the disturbing sensation of living life on a treadmill, a life with no rest. Struggling to keep up *and* keep going, the need to *do* is driven by an overwhelming sense that if we *were* to stop, everything would somehow fall apart, and that we would have failed, somehow, in life.

In those moments before we do finally collapse into bed, we often use TV, food, and alcohol to help us unwind while we keep our fingers crossed that *this* is the week our lottery numbers will come up and we'll finally get that dream holiday (and with it the chance to relax). Until that happens, if our relaxation depends on watching violent or psychological thrillers before bed or endless Netflix with its seductive "one more episode …" teaser, than rather than relax we continue to stimulate the brain further. Likewise if late night snacking is our comfort, we ask the digestive system to keep working, and if alcohol is our go-to, we may find that those few glasses of red before bed disrupts our sleeping patterns. It's not that you have to give up these pleasures, but instead realise that eating, drinking, and watching TV stimulates our system, and so while fine in their own space, they do not actually count as forms of rest.

The reward we are offered in return for our constant activity is the badge of busyness. Despite the fact that we live in an age of technology promising to help us to get more done in less time, it seems that we are trying to use all our time to do more. We still dash around trying to fit in an extra coffee, an extra meeting, an extra gym class—and often find ourselves validated for it. Our society celebrates the "work hard, play hard" attitude that dominates our politics, media, and culture, but an overload of activity often leads to burnout as our bodies and brains try to keep up with a pace of life which we simply weren't built for. Instead of thriving in the advance of technology, many of us feel that we are (barely) surviving, and that somehow, we're to blame.

Many of us have woken up to the detriment that our continuous activity has on our health and well-being, and the surge of popularity in yoga is no doubt due to more and more people looking for ways to de-stress and relax. As we increase our understanding of the mind-body connection, the need for "another way" becomes greater and this is where yoga comes in. Yoga, known for its relaxing and stress-relieving benefits, is now a billion dollar industry. In 2017 the yoga market was reckoned to be worth $16bn (£12bn) in the US and $80bn (£74bn) globally,[3] and in the UK, "yoga" was one of Google's most searched-for words in 2016. But despite spending millions on "super" foods, expen-sive gym memberships, and pretty yoga clothes, our tiredness just isn't going away.

It is my hope that this book will help you to understand not only why rest is radical, but how to reclaim your right to rest. When the soci-etal values of constant striving and pushing are widely applauded as symbols of success, it takes courage to slow down and honour our need to rest, but it's not a dramatisation to say that our health, happiness, and future may depend on it. Not only do many of us long for change in our personal lives, but collectively there is growing desire to change the way we treat our Earth. Ugly buildings, lack of green space, cruelty to animals, polluted air, and plastic in our seas—the time has come for us to realise that this chapter in history is coming to an end. What will we discover when we turn the page? I don't have the answer to that, but I do know that when we feel tired, numb, and powerless, the thought of tackling the washing-up can feel too much, let alone the problems of the world.

All of that is about to change. By learning how to nurture and nour-ish your body and mind through the simple act of rest, you will begin to see just how you can change your life, and the world around you, for the better. We are in this together. Your energy matters, you matter.

You *can* be the change you want to see in the world by making that change in your own life. The best thing of all about Radical Rest is that it mostly involves lying down, but before that, let me tell you more about this book.

About this book

This is a book which highlights the power of Radical Rest as a tool for better health but also as a way to see yourself and the world beyond the physical and material. It introduces the concept of resting as a radical act to all those who are ready for another way, to those who are looking to find a little more harmony in their daily lives and rediscover a love and joy for the life they have right now (not the life they hope for in ten years' time). This book is for those looking to make long-lasting change to the way that they live, but want it in bite-size pieces.

This book offers a practical guide to rest. It is written for busy people with busy lives, people with families and jobs and other responsibilities. It doesn't demand unrealistic changes on your part, or suggest a ten-step plan to success; rather it tempts you into finding ways to rest more in your day-to-day life, to make life feel more easeful and peaceful without drastic effort on your part. No need to lose weight, no need to twist yourself into a pretzel-like position or stand on your head, no: this book is for real people with real lives, who could see their health, relationships, and work improve radically by taking more rest. This book frames practical suggestions with research and insight, it combines stories of triumph over adversity with a sprinkle of philosophical yogic ponderings, and most of all it aims to encourage you, the reader, to consider if Radical Rest could improve your life.

This is not a textbook, an instruction manual, or a scientific paper. It is a book of stories, of sharing, of hope and (hopefully) some humour. I share my own personal experiences as well as sharing the stories of those I have worked with in my role as a yoga teacher. I define any suffering from stress, anxiety, addiction, depression, grief, trauma, or menstrual health as "calls to rest," the symptoms of an overworked mind, stressed-out body, and neglected soul, and explore these complex issues from the viewpoint of Radical Rest. I don't believe in a one-size-fits-all answer, so while my intention is to highlight and celebrate the power of resting with you, I also draw upon the research and teachings of others to add new perspectives and insights. My deepest gratitude goes to some of my favourite authors and teachers, who are listed in the reading list at the end of this book.

I invite you to take what you need from this book, be it practical tips and ideas for reducing stress or the more radical notion that we are spiritual creatures and this system in which we find ourselves was built for machines, not beautiful creative human beings. I support the idea that we are souls and within our tired and achy bodies and our frazzled minds there is something whole, complete, and perfect, but if this idea seems a bit too extreme or airy-fairy for you, you can put it to one side and focus purely on the practical.

What is Radical Rest?

Radical Rest is a form of active, conscious rest achieved primarily through the practices of restorative yoga and yoga nidra and the application of the principles that define it. This is yoga but not as you know it. Radical Rest requires no expensive equipment, no 4am starts and no pilgrimages to India. It is for all genders, all ages, all shapes, colours, and sizes. It simply requires you to make the time and space to reconnect with your deepest, wisest self—all through resting. There are nine principles to Radical Rest: compassion, curiosity, creativity, caution, courage, community, connection, consciousness, and finally, contemplation. All of these principles are designed to help you bring more aspects of Radical Rest into your daily life, and we will delve more deeply into those principles in the next chapter.

Where did it come from?

The inspiration for this book came when I was attending a unique and intensive yoga nidra course on the wild Aran Islands, on the west coast of Ireland in 2016; more on this in the next chapter. In Chapter 4 I also share a brief history and background of restorative yoga and yoga nidra, which make the bedrock of Radical Rest, and how I came to be writing this book.

What are restorative yoga and yoga nidra?

Restorative yoga is a deeply relaxing form of yoga practice. In restorative yoga, we use soothing "asana" (postures) in which the body is fully supported by props like yoga bolsters and blankets. Many of the poses are performed lying still. This means that rather than having to make an effort, you can sink into the postures to release tension and achieve deep relaxation.

Yoga nidra is a guided meditation practice that is simple yet often profoundly beneficial. It involves lying down in a comfortable position, and being guided through a meditation which deeply relaxes the body, and unlike other meditation, there's no effort needed—you can't get it wrong! By combining both restorative yoga and yoga nidra, we bring great relaxation to the body and mind. Chapter 4 is dedicated to exploring restorative yoga and yoga nidra in more depth.

Why yoga?

Yoga is a philosophy which uses physical practices such as postures, breathing, and meditation as ways to wake up our individual and universal consciousness. Through yoga we become more "awake" and are able to take more responsibility over our lives, as well as to develop greater sensitivity and understanding. Yoga is also a fully integrated system, involving mind, body, and soul, and feeds each layer of our being whenever we practise. There are many types of yoga and many ways to practise, from the more common hatha yoga which uses posture work, breathing techniques, and meditation as a way to purify the body, to bhakti yoga which uses chanting and devotional singing techniques.

What about other types of yoga?

Although I love all the many diverse ways to practise yoga, this book aims to highlight these gentle and compassionate yoga practices as pathways towards deep acceptance and love. It showcases the softer side to yoga, the restorative and contemplative side which sometimes gets shunned in favour of "workout" yoga. Although not physically demanding, the practices of restorative yoga and yoga nidra offer the power to transform our well-being and our lives precisely by doing less, not more. It is for all those who feel lost on the path of yoga, as well as all those who have been put off from trying yoga out of fears of not being good/slim/young/flexible enough. You do not need to be a yogi in order to benefit from this book—in fact you don't need to have ever practised yoga. You may however wish to get advice from your doctor before taking on any of the practices that I mention, particularly if you have any physical or mental health conditions, past or present.

Who is this book for?

This is a book for anyone who has felt sick and tired of feeling sick and tired; anyone who longs for another way beyond deadlines and to-do lists; anyone who is ready for an easy way to feel better—anyone who is ready to make simple changes to their life to improve their physical, mental, and emotional well-being. It is for men and women, although there is a section specifically on the menstrual cycle due to the increasing number of women experiencing difficulties in this area and the link between women's health and the cycles of the Earth.

This book is for you if you are:

- Feeling exhausted, disconnected, or numb
- Burnt out
- Feeling overwhelmed by environmental/political/social situations
- Suffering with menstrual/fertility health problems (or living with someone who is)
- Out of contact with your creativity and joy for living
- Looking for a refreshing approach to spirituality and yoga
- Anyone who has simply forgotten how to rest
- And any or all of the above!

How to use this book

You might want to read this book in a good old-fashioned way from beginning to end, or you may feel inclined to delve into a chapter which feels relevant for you right now.

In Chapters 6 to 12, I will look at stress, anxiety, addiction, depression, grief, trauma, and menstrual health under the headline "calls to rest," sharing stories from my own personal experiences as well as those from students I work with, some contemporary and philosophical thoughts, and practical advice on how to practise restorative yoga postures at home, as well as information on where to find yoga nidra recordings. I also share breathing exercises that may help you, so if you're experiencing one of these conditions and want to get started then you might want to skip straight to the relevant section—please do read the chapter preceding the "calls to rest," entitled "You have been called to rest" as this chapter offers some useful preparatory advice as well as some precautions. I choose these topics as they are all areas in which I have had personal and professional experience, and so my study and practice have evolved around my attempts to heal myself, and also to support clients on their own healing journeys.

If you're looking for more practical things to get you started straight away, check out the Radical Rest toolbox at the end of the book, where you can explore tools beyond restorative yoga, breathing practices, and yoga nidra to become a Radical Restivist. Towards the end of the book I go back to my own story and journey into Radical Rest, as well as recommend resources for a more restful life.

If you need more convincing about the importance of rest in our lives, check out Chapter 3, where I share some facts about the changes in our sleep and napping culture, and the impact this is having. In the next chapter, I introduce restorative yoga and yoga nidra, and why they are such an asset to the stressed-out, tired-out person. I also explain why resting can be a spiritual practice—if approached in the right way. If you prefer to continue straight from here you will find a very different story of my life ten years ago, as well as the story of how Radical Rest was born, and read more about the nine principles of Radical Rest. There is no right or wrong way to read or explore this book so sit back and dive in.

About me

I am a yoga teacher, reflexologist, writer (this book, blogs, and occasional poetry), and a lover of yoga, particularly restorative yoga and yoga nidra. I became a qualified yoga teacher in 2014, and launched into intensive study, both with a number of skilled and inspirational teachers and alone with a yoga mat and plenty of books. In that time I discovered more about myself than I would have thought possible. I became aware of the link between my mental and physical well-being and the unresolved grief of losing my caregivers and home (all before the age of eighteen) that I had been carrying for my entire adult life. I woke up to the fact that my oh-so-important career was burning me out. I learnt a new way to listen to my body and I started to explore new ways to live my life, and I began to think about what it means to trust in a higher power. Along the way I realised the importance of learning to trust myself, which required respecting and loving myself first. This will probably be my lifelong practice.

In recent years my understanding and awareness has been deepened by attempting to live the ideology behind *Rest Is Radical* and I am honoured to teach classes, workshops, and retreats to groups and to work one-to-one with a variety of clients suffering with anxiety, PTSD, depression, stress, low self-esteem, and more. I have specialised my training in restorative yoga, yoga nidra, and yoga for women's wellbeing (although I love to practise all forms of yoga), and I am fascinated by the body's capacity to heal itself, and the potential held within the mind. I have read a lot of books, I track my menstrual cycle, I journal, and most of what I have learnt has come from my own lived experience.

I love to study and am looking forward to where my studies take me next—currently astrology and philosophy. I live in Bristol with my husband who is an artist and despite the unpredictability of our being yogis and artists, I am grateful for the creativity in our lives. I am also deeply grateful to yoga for leading me to the pathway of Radical Rest, which undoubtedly has radically changed my life, and I am excited to pass on what I have so far learnt to you in this book. I am most grateful to the people who show up to class, to a one-to-one session, or a workshop or retreat. I learn so much from them, and they are my biggest motivation.

CHAPTER TWO

Gifted

Tired, busy, stressed: these words summed up my life ten years ago, when going above and beyond at work was my way of proving myself in the world and avoiding my grief. I was exhausted, wondering how bad things had to get before I could officially say I was burnt out, yet I still continued to push myself hard with little time for rest. Everyone around me seemed to be tired, stressed, and busy, why should I be any different? Feeling short-tempered, irritable, unhappy, and overwhelmed felt like a natural response to most situations, and my forays into depression and anxiety became more frequent while my physical health seemed to be weakening despite the miles I clocked up on my morning runs or the hours at the gym after work.

Starting a yoga teachers' training course had already begun to change my perspective on the world, but it wasn't until a five day yoga nidra retreat that I discovered what it meant to completely relax and let go. This was the start of something big, but of course, like everyone else, after the retreat I had to return to a busy diary and demanding job. I did however start to practise yoga nidra at least once a day. I went on to train in restorative yoga, and felt such relief from the technique that for a while it became my main yoga practice. It wasn't until three years later, when I had given up my career and become a full-time yoga teacher, that I was "given" the idea of *Rest Is Radical*.

I was on another yoga nidra course, this time on Inishmore, one of the wild Aran Islands on the rugged and often fierce west Irish coast. Yoga nidra is, as I briefly mentioned in the introduction to this book, an incredibly profound and transformative meditation practice which I will discuss in more detail in Chapter 4. Collectively we were taking this practice perhaps eleven plus times a day, with no outside distractions and just the roaring Atlantic Ocean and remote limestone cliffs to keep us company. This was certainly a unique environment to be in, and one which I am sure helped the idea of *Rest Is Radical* be born.

One evening after listening to captivating pagan stories from Celtic priest Dara Molloy I felt full of energy, and was compelled to hike to the top of Dún Aonghasa (pronounced Dung Angus). Dún Aonghasa is very impressive. It's an amphitheatre-like fort resting on the edge of a 300 foot sheer drop to nothing but the wild Atlantic Ocean. We'd visited Dún Aonghasa as a group, with some of us choosing to go up there early in the morning for yoga practice. It always felt wild no matter what time of day, but at 10pm in midsummer it certainly felt wilder than ever. Reaching the top, I decided to do something I hadn't been brave enough to do before—lie on my stomach and shuffle my head over the edge at the 300 foot sheer drop to the ocean and rocks. Alone and at night, it was exhilarating. After hovering my camera with somewhat trembling hands over the edge, and taking a few snaps, I pulled myself back. Lifting myself up and off my stomach was almost as terrifying as looking down! I was trembling, my heart was racing, energy coursed through my body and I felt awake and alive. I started to make my way back down the cliff when suddenly, it came to me: *rest is radical*.

It was like someone or something whispering into my ear. It was as though the land were speaking to me. I didn't feel like I had come up with a slogan or catchphrase, and at that moment I didn't even really know what the words meant. But the Earth's voice was whispering, *rest is radical, rest is radical*, and I somehow knew that I was being asked to do something. I love the words of poet John O'Donohue, "You have travelled too fast over false ground/now your soul has come, to take you back."[1] These words felt so pertinent not only to my own life but to the lives of so many people I knew. Yoga had awakened me to the concept of the soul, and now was the time to explore what it took to live a soul-full life.

In her book *Big Magic*, Elizabeth Gilbert talks about ideas as never belonging to us. She describes them as visiting us, asking us to take action, and when we don't, they shoot off elsewhere, usually somewhere close to home, which is why when an idea comes to us and we don't act on it, we often see someone else nearby doing the same thing, taking action on what we had considered "our" idea.[2] This was exactly how I felt—this wasn't my idea but this idea had chosen to come to me, at that place, at that moment. I made a promise there and then to do the work, despite not knowing what the work was going to be.

This was a gift. Through the wild landscape of the Aran Islands, Dara Molloy's evocative storytelling, yoga teacher Uma Dinsmore-Tuli's creative teachings, and the practice of yoga nidra itself, I was gifted with the task of sharing "rest is radical"—once I knew what it was! This book puts onto paper my research but also my personal experiences and understanding of what it means to take conscious rest, and what makes this so radical. A very big part of my work was to actually figure out how to rest myself. That was the hard bit and at the end of this book, I share with you my own personal, heartfelt account of how I experienced rest. It wasn't always easy, but it certainly was radical.

So what is Radical Rest? I have defined it as:

> **Radical Rest** (adjective, noun, and verb):
> *healing, conscious rest to return us to our forgotten state of deep relaxation primarily through the practice of restorative yoga and yoga nidra.*

The foundation of Radical Rest comes in the nine following principles. Although these principles form the basis of the ideology behind Radical Rest, anything that is radical cannot be defined in a neat and tidy list of nine (even if they do all conveniently begin with the letter C). However, these principles are designed to help you implement the practice of Radical Rest.

1. Compassion

Compassion is an essential tool to have in our lives and plays a big role in a lot of spiritual practices, including yoga and Buddhism. Without it we become hard, and our relationships suffer, including the relationship with our own self. Compassion helps us to understand that making change is difficult, and so we don't give ourselves a hard time if we struggle in our journey towards rest, perhaps falling back into old patterns or negative thinking. Our empathy with ourselves and others makes resting more possible as we grow to fully understand that we have a real need to rest. As we start to respect and respond to that need, so we allow others to voice their need to rest, thus increasing our capacity for compassion and kindness as we recognise our limits and our expectations of others. Importantly, we are able to forgive ourselves for our need to slow down and become more accepting of who we truly are.

2. Curiosity

Remain open-minded at all times. This book is not set in stone, and neither are these principles. You may find new ways that help you to radically rest or you may disagree with sections of the book, or have a new perspective to offer. I welcome and encourage your curiosity and debate. Radical Rest is designed to change the way we have been conditioned to think and act, to step into new and perhaps uncharted territory. Be open to what comes your way, and remain curious, not competitive, about your experiences. Our feelings usually want to be acknowledged and expressed. Radical Rest teaches us how to become more curious and less critical of our experiences, which allows us to avoid getting trapped in any dogmatic thought patterns that can actually hinder our development. In the same way that what you desired when you were twenty-one is probably different to what you desire aged sixty-one, your methods of resting are very likely to change throughout your lifetime. Curiosity is a way to retain an open mind and feel young-at-heart as you go through life.

3. Creativity

This is a creative process, and creativity goes hand in hand with principle two, curiosity. As you learn to trust more fully in your intuition, you may find the way you practise Radical Rest begins to change. After years of very still practice, I found myself drawn to free dance, which whilst energetic left me feeling nourished and relaxed. After many years of dedicated yoga nidra practice, I have been able to make more of my daily life restful so I am not as exhausted as I was before, and other activities can be replenishing to me. Remember these are tools to support you and empower you in your daily life; they are not designed to hinder your progress, frustrate you, or become another joyless regime.

4. Caution

Any personal or spiritual work takes time. Habits must be made, life-styles amended, and so I include caution as a reminder to manage your expectations. Trying to make drastic changes in your life can be difficult or even impossible, and you may find yourself becoming disheartened and disillusioned. Bear in mind that when you allow your body to return to its own natural rhythm, you may have times when you feel more tired. At first this can be demotivating and even alarming, but it is often simply our body's natural ebb and flow of energy. Caution is also needed if you are suffering from a trauma of some kind. In this case, you may prefer to practise yoga nidra with an experienced teacher in a one-to-one setting or find a sympathetic counsellor or psychotherapist to support you. One size does not fit all. Trust yourself, invest in your practice, and remember that Rome wasn't built in a day.

5. Courage

After the slightly saturnine warning of caution above, time to bring in the courage. Oh courage, our beloved companion so needed during these times of crisis and upheaval. Courage comes from our heart and we embrace courage every day we choose to persevere with our heart's desire, despite the warnings and nay-saying from those around us (and the nay-sayer in our very own head). Courage comes when we dare to be ourselves, however odd, eccentric, or just plain weird we deem that to be. To have courage to relax sounds odd, but in a life that never stops, with phones which never turn off, to drop down tools and simply just *be* can take courage. We are often our most courageous when we feel the most vulnerable, when we're not really sure we can do it after all, yet we continue to tentatively move forward onto less familiar ground. It's a gift we all possess but it's a gift that we must cultivate, look for, and welcome in.

6. Community

Courage is often a solo endeavour and so having a support network can be the difference between making long-lasting changes in your life and becoming disillusioned and giving up. Look for restorative yoga and yoga nidra teachers near you. Share this book with a friend and see if they want to be your "rest-ie best-ie" (or words to that effect). Ask your local library to stock it, or start a book club. You don't need to get rid of all your "work hard, play hard" friends, but start to consider if you could benefit from new friendships with those who also yearn to live a more restful life, as well as adding elements of restfulness to existing friendships by suggesting calmer ways to spend time together. They might just need permission to rest, as so many of us do.

7. Connection

Slightly different to community, which is about making outward con-nections, this is about your connection inward. This is what the practices of Radical Rest can bring us, the chance to visit the internal landscape of thoughts, feelings, and beliefs and to discover the real peace that lies within. It is this journey to a world beyond the ordinary, this encounter with the Divine that ultimately becomes our true motivation. Medita-tion of any kind including yoga nidra is the practice of quietening the ego and accessing the Divine nature that resides both within us and without us. It is only through stillness that we experience this—and Radical Rest makes this almost effortless, as by relaxing first the body, we are truly able to relax the mind.

8. Consciousness

Becoming more conscious simply means to increase our awareness and become responsive rather than reactive. Scientific studies are show-ing that regular meditation practice can increase the parts of the brain that deal with both cognitive and emotional processing, making us less reactive to stress, more tolerant to difficult situations, and providing us with clearer thoughts. This helps us begin to see ourselves as some-thing beyond the everyday stresses and worries, beyond our identities as workers, parents, or friends, and instead understand ourselves in a much fuller, and deeper way. Practically speaking, relaxing muscle tension creates space in the body for the breath which reduces stress, increases our feelings of calm, and helps us become more capable in responding to the situations that we face.

9. Contemplation

Contemplation is a form of wisdom that helps us explore and consider the world around us as well as the meaning of our own existence. The more we begin to recognise and experience ourselves as more than physical beings, even if we don't have the words or sentiments to express that recognition, the more we relax into who we truly are. Contemplation is a profound form of thought that is beyond the general chit-chat of the mind, a deeper and more soulful way of thinking, less concerned with exact answers and rhetoric and more concerned with the expansion of the human mind beyond the need to survive, and more towards true meaning and philosophy. When we practise Radical Rest we open ourselves to the possibility of contemplation. We find ourselves craving more time alone, more quiet, less noise and distraction, and when this starts to happen (which it will, you don't need to force it), you are entering into the sacred art of contemplation. Enjoy!

These are principles which I will refer back to throughout the book. They are by their very nature evolving, open to critique and change, and wonderful topics to contemplate on. They add an element of depth to the practice of Radical Rest, a depth which is inherent in yoga but perhaps not always so easily expressed in a sixty minute yoga class. They are thoughts, ponderings, ideas that I still reflect on now. But before we get too lost in philosophical concepts, let's come back to earth for a moment and explore: how is it that we need Radical Rest—just how did we get so radically tired?

CHAPTER THREE

Ready to rest

Ah, sleep. Surely one of life's greatest pleasures, yet how many of us feel we are sleeping as well and as much as we would like? Apparently not many of us, as reports on the subject agree that the quality and quantity of our sleep is in decline. The Sleep Council's Great British Bedtime Report of 2017[1] showed that we are getting less sleep than in 2013, due to stress and worry (the third reason being partner disturbance—sorry to be a romance-killer).

Stats and facts prove what we already know: sleep matters. Whether you want to have glowing skin, to burn off the extra piece of cake you snuck in, or just to properly rest your body from the labours of the day, you're going to need to get into bed and go to sleep early my friends because that brain of yours has got *a lot* of processing to do in these precious hours. All that scrolling through social media or inboxes? That heart-stopping moment when you stepped off the pavement and into a speeding cyclist? The news you've consumed, the pavements you've pounded, the busy schedule you've been negotiating—the brain has got a lot to work on while you're getting your beauty sleep and it's not going to get everything done in five hours of restless, agitated sleep.

Even within the yoga philosophy conceived in a very different lifetime (one without smartphones and climate change to contend with)

21

it was thought that going to bed tense created a tense sleep, which could explain why many of us wake up feeling tired. How much sleep we need changes. Sometimes we get it, sometimes not (I'm still talking about sleep here ...). If you work shifts, have kids, or simply don't sleep well do not worry about it. First of all, when did worrying ever help anything? And second, although the meme of the moment dictates we should all be getting eight hours of solid sleep per night, prior to Industrialisation it was not uncommon for people to wake in the middle of the night, perhaps smoke a cigarette, gossip with a neighbour, or (something still familiar to many of us) pop to the loo, before returning to their slumber.

Waking in the night was not always considered a problem, whereas now we are often bombarded with scary headlines and ever changing statistics about what might happen if we neglect our sleep, ironically increasing anxiety over getting the perfect night's sleep and leading to higher rates of insomnia. Keep calm and read on! Rather than save up resting just for night time, this book invites you to consider making your days more restful and in doing so, making life more restful. If sleep is eluding you, then it becomes more useful to find a way to restore yourself in the day time. One way to do this is to nap.

The importance of taking naps

Humans have a circadian rhythm which means that we often feel our energy drop some point in the afternoon. This is the body's way of telling us that we must rest in order to get through the remainder of the day before bedtime, yet many of us find ourselves at work or out and about, with an inconvenient lack of beds at our disposal. You may scoff at the idea of naps or believe naps are exclusively for the use of babies and sick people. And while naps are not for everyone, our cultural attitude to napping no doubt goes along with the decline in recognition and appreciation for rest in general.

The rise of industrialism saw more people move to cities and towns working in places like factories and away from more agricultural work on the land, changing the dynamic not only in how we work but also changing the intimacy of our relationship with nature. No longer needing to pay attention to season changes, to shifts in light and temperature, humans were able to work in shifts, to someone else's clock. I'm not romanticising agricultural working or labelling industrialisation as the bad guy here (for one I'm not a historian so I don't know enough facts and two I don't find it helpful to look back at the "good old days" with too much wistfulness and nostalgia), but simply drawing a very basic historical backdrop to the sleep patterns today where many people are finding they barely have enough time for sleeping, let alone consider napping. Work and the deceptively aspirational banner of productivity trumps all else and even though huge global corporates like Google and Nike apparently have nap rooms for employees, this is most likely only due to the understanding that napping encourages productivity. While being more productive can be useful, the aim of this book is not to make you more productive but to help you acknowledge and respond to your need to rest *just because you need to*.

Each of us is, of course, programmed uniquely, and what works for one might not work for another. The more we can understand our own individual needs, the easier it becomes to understand how much sleep we need, and just how and when to nap. Recognise that the need to nap and the desire to lay down tools throughout the day is not a problem to be fixed but simply a message from our body asking us to respond. In the way we need to eat and drink, we also need to rest. Many of us (myself included) frequently experience the so-called afternoon slump, but for many of us the idea or possibility of following the urge to lie down and nap just isn't feasible, and anyway, we're also drawn to the thought of coffee and sugar to keep us going. If you could lie down and nap, would you? Or would you prefer to keep pushing through? While the ability to be plugged in and working around the clock certainly contribute to our increasing lack of rest, I believe it can be a valuable exercise to reflect on your own feelings and beliefs about taking rest.

Let's say you have a window of opportunity. The stars align to give you the time, place, and space to nap. You even manage to convince that slave driver mind of yours to remember all the benefits in resting, including those USPs of greater productivity, creativity, and physical restoration. You lie down, and wait to feel rested. But your mind is buzzing, you feel restless. Suddenly you need a drink of water, you feel too hot, or too cold. You remember that email you've been meaning to reply to, and before you know it you are back at your laptop typing furiously away. Even if you resist the urge to respond to any of those desires, you simply lie there feeling frustrated and bored and wondering why on earth you decided to try this napping thing in the first place.

When we are removed from our natural rhythms and when we are used to finding ways to push through, it's not always easy to simply introduce new tactics and expect them to work straight away. The more stressed or wired we are, the harder we might find it to rest as the stress hormones careering through the body continue to pump through our veins in preparation for the next potential crisis. Equally, it may be that we are keeping ourselves busy for a reason, staying distracted to avoid actually listening to our thoughts and feelings for fear that they may be uncomfortable or unpleasant. It may be easier to reach for the smartphone than it is to simply keep yourself company, and so lying down and doing nothing may feel impossible. If any of the above sounds like you, then what can you do?

Radical Rest, of course.

Radical Rest is, you may remember, a form of healing, conscious rest primarily experienced through the practices of restorative yoga and yoga nidra. For those of us who cannot bring ourselves to nap, or just find napping impossible, Radical Rest helps us to create an environment to make resting easier. Your body is the environment, and so by relaxing the body you can quickly feel calmer and more content. Radical Rest actively holds the body in yoga postures with no muscular effort. Let me say that again—no muscular effort. Nope, no standing on your head or putting your foot to your ear required here. No sweating, no Lycra, and no flat bellies. In fact, the softer the belly, the better, because this means that the muscle tension is releasing and you will be able to breathe more fully and deeply, an essential part of stress reduction and a key component of Radical Rest. We are better able to respond, to choose what action to take in that moment, and that might make lying down for twenty minutes much more feasible than if we're pumped up on adrenaline and stress. We practise Radical Rest through two forms of yoga techniques, restorative yoga and yoga nidra, and in the next chapter I will guide you through each of these techniques and introduce you to yoga, just not as you know it.

CHAPTER FOUR

The tools

R eading this book about rest is a great place to start, but to fully understand the power of rest we must embody it. In the fields of yoga, bodywork, and movement therapies there is great talk about the mind-body connection, but outside those fields you'd be forgiven for thinking that the mind and the body have nothing to do with one another. If we have a problem with our body, we don't often pause to consider if our mental or emotional health may have played a role in the physical problem. How many of us, when faced with tense shoulders for example, stop to ask ourselves if we are holding onto old heartbreak, carrying too much responsibility, or indeed, carrying the weight of the world on those shoulders?

It might sound strange to begin with. Many of us were brought up with the idea that the doctor always knows best, and that when there is a problem to take a pill and wait for a cure. While there is no doubt that the allopathic medical world has made huge leaps and bounds in the diagnosis and treatment of certain illnesses, this science-based modern approach does often miss out the integral connection between the way we live, think, and act out our lives with our physical well-being. The mind-body connection is based on the belief that there is a relationship between the body and mind and that this relationship directly impacts

25

our sense of health and well-being. An easy example is to think of a time when you felt very nervous, perhaps taking your driving test, or sitting for an important exam. You may have needed to go to the toilet more frequently, or felt nauseous. This is an example of how the thoughts in the mind impact the experience of being in our bodies, but at any given time our emotions and thoughts can affect our physical being because they are part of our physical being.

Yoga helps us to understand the mind-body connection by asking us to bring both together in our yoga practice. Whether we are attempting to breathe and move in synchronicity, or stay focused on our thoughts during a meditation practice, we are usually trying to calm the body through engaging the mind, or still the mind by releasing tension from the body. Although yoga can have a reputation for being a very physical practice, it actually has many methods and techniques to it, which can be made suitable for everybody. Certainly when it comes to restorative yoga and yoga nidra there is no need to contort yourself into pretzel-like positions, and you don't need to be able to touch your toes, balance on one leg, or wear a certain dress size. Whilst it is always recommended that you consult your doctor or health professional before embarking on a new exercise programme, particularly if you are pregnant, recovering from surgery, or have an existing health condition, on the whole, restorative yoga and yoga nidra are for everybody. There is no need to already be flexible or fit, in fact there is no requirement for any particular skill at yoga postures at all—what a relief!

Restorative yoga and yoga nidra are true tonics for our stressed-out, worn out, anxious times as they teach us (or perhaps we might say *remind* us) how to relax. Together, they create the perfect setting for deep, radical rest. I have been practising both restorative yoga and yoga nidra for years now, and I am still amazed by the refreshing quality of both techniques. In this chapter I will share more about why the practices are so restful, as well as sharing some historical context. My aim is to share just enough information to give you a deeper understanding of how these types of yoga can benefit body, mind, and breath, and just why this is so wonderfully restful.

Restorative yoga

Let's start with restorative yoga. I can't remember exactly when I first came to restorative yoga, but I do remember that it gradually took over as my main form of practice. As a yoga teacher and advocate of conscious rest I generally practise some form of restful meditative movement each day but it isn't essential that you need to start a daily practice. You may find the more Radical Rest you experience, the better it makes you feel, and so you want to do more, but certainly at the start, one session a week could make all the difference.

A very brief history ...

Restorative yoga in itself is a relatively modern interpretation of yoga. While the exact origins of yoga is a controversial point (with some researchers and scholars believing it to be around 5000 years old, and others believing it is older than that again), restorative yoga is a more recent form of yoga practice, developed very much for the ailments of our times. Developed most famously by Judith Hanson Lasater, an American yoga teacher who trained with B. K. S. Iyengar (you may have heard of Iyengar yoga, named after the Indian teacher), it has grown in popularity as more people catch on to the idea of a form of exercise which is also deeply restful. Unlike other forms of yoga, restorative yoga is very much focused on softening the muscles of the body rather than strengthening or stretching. Whilst other forms of yoga can also be relaxing, they are not always suitable for those who are injured, ill, menstruating, pregnant, or fatigued. Restorative yoga can be complementary to more energetic forms of yoga practice, but it can also be the focus of one's practice, depending on the individual's needs.

By using a lot of yoga equipment (usually called yoga props) to hold the body in certain postures designed to reduce feelings of stress, it is a slow practice, with postures usually being held for somewhere between two minutes and as much as forty-five minutes at a time, and unlike other forms of yoga practice, restorative yoga focuses purely on relaxation. Restorative yoga can be practised by most people, regardless of flexibility or strength. All the postures are performed lying down, and the use of props means that there is little, if any, muscular effort.

By completely relaxing the body in this way, we are able to dissolve mental as well as physical agitation. Remember the mind-body connection? Well, by resting the body in postures designed to activate the parasympathetic nervous system (the part of the brain responsible for keeping us calm and relaxed), we are engaging with the mind-body connection, calming the mind to relax the body, relaxing the body to calm the mind. This will be explained more fully in the chapter on stress, but for now know that restorative yoga is very good for your health!

Restorative yoga is different from simply napping or just lying down. Restorative yoga helps us to relax the body more quickly and more deeply through the nature of the postures that we take. For example, we may take a face-down posture, such as a child's pose (see page 68) if we want to quiet the mind and take our attention inward. If we are fatigued we may want to gently re-energise, for example taking the legs up against the wall (see page 105) in order to encourage blood flow back down to the heart and let go of the fight with gravity. There is always a posture designed for our needs, and I will go into this in more detail in the coming chapters entitled Calls to Rest.

When teaching classes or workshops, I often remind students that this is a type of yoga which will help us increase our *emotional* strength, rather than our *physical* strength. It can however complement other forms of more vigorous yoga practices we may be doing, by encouraging muscles to lengthen, release, soften, and create more space. When we fully relax the body, we are also relaxing the breath. If you imagine for a moment the posture you hold while sitting at your laptop, or hunched over your phone, you can see how the chest is collapsed, the upper back rounded, jaw tense, and shoulders tight. This posture does not provide the optimal position for the lungs to breathe fully and deeply, for the rib cage to expand and the intercostal muscles to stretch. When we hold the physical body in this way, we limit our ability to take full and deep breaths.

In comparison, by opening up the chest, lengthening the abdomen, and creating space for our natural breath to emerge, we are naturally encouraging the breath to become fuller and deeper, which in turn invites the mind to slow down, and become more steady and calm. This is an example of how yoga understands and supports the mind-body connection. Breath is a very important part of our yoga practice, and is wonderfully accessible to everyone, including beginners. If you can breathe, you can do yoga! Breath is essential to the optimal functioning of your body, from your heart and lungs to your digestive organs and even the brain.

If you feel that you are struggling to keep up with the fast pace of life, your breath may feel the same. Chronic stress and bad posture can result in unhealthy breath patterns, so anything that we can do to improve our sense of relaxation will greatly improve the quality of our breath and vice versa. If in times of worry we can remember to pause and take some slow, deep breaths, we can instantly notice how much calmer we feel. Our problems may not have gone away, but we have improved our ability to respond to those problems in a more logical and helpful way, rather than perhaps reacting out of panic or fear.

Restorative yoga helps to create space for the breath by gently opening the muscles which are essential for our natural breath and yet are common areas of tension, including in places like the jaw, neck, shoulders, diaphragm, hips, and legs. Not only does restorative yoga encourage the body to open like a flower towards the sun, the fact we have removed all effort can be hugely beneficial to the mind, particularly for those who find that they need to stay active and productive all the time (and I myself often fall into this camp). By embodying what it is to relax, we find it easier to return to this state time and time again. This is why restorative yoga, like all forms of yoga practice, are more effective when practised frequently, and in later chapters I will be sharing with you some of my favourite postures that you can try at home.

Letting go, seeing clearly

For those of us more familiar to pushing ourselves hard, learning to let go of effort can sometimes be a difficult idea to get our heads around. I sometimes notice students ignoring instructions to avoid any active stretching and instead become aware of a more gentle and less obvious sense of letting go, perhaps out of habit or belief that to push harder is to achieve more, which is not the case within Radical Rest. The temptation to push harder and to try to feel something can be difficult to resist, particularly if we are having a hard time relaxing in life. Luckily restorative yoga is designed to calm us down, meaning we find being still much easier than we had imagined. It can take time for us to relax deeply, and this might not happen the first time we practise restorative yoga. One thing that can happen is we may become more aware of our aches and pains. This is not a reason to give up on the practice or to stop, it merely shows that the practice is working, as we are becoming more aware of our body and its sensations, as well as increasing our capacity to be able to stay present in the face of discomfort. This is an invaluable tool, particularly if you find yourself turning on the TV or browsing the internet in times of difficulty or angst.

One of the great teachings of yoga as well as of other spiritual practices like Buddhism is to be able to acknowledge that there is suffering in the world. If we are able to practise being aware of an ache in our lower back or tightness in the jaw, for example, then we are also practising how to be present in the face of the suffering we see in the world, on the streets around us, and also in the images presented to us via the media. It may seem like a big stretch at first to go from relaxing your body to being present in the face of suffering, but if we think of Radical Rest as an awakening, we can understand that part of that awakening involves seeing the pain in the world as well as the beauty. This is where our fifth principle of courage comes into practice.

I often describe restorative yoga as a gateway to meditation because it teaches us to embody stillness and silence, two key components of meditation practice. It also teaches us to be comfortable with spending time with our thoughts, away from our phones and other distractions. It becomes a form of meditation as we are able to "watch" the mind in its frantic leaping from one thought to the next. This is sometimes known as observing the mind, and in being able to observe the mind we are able to take appropriate action, rather than reacting out of fear or anxiety. For example, if we watch the news repeatedly throughout the day, and we start to notice that we are often holding the breath or that we are constantly worrying, we may proactively take the choice to stop watching the news quite so much. We take conscious action through our observation.

We may also become aware of repetitive thought patterns we have, or beliefs that we hold about ourselves or the world, and with that awareness, we are able to reflect on whether those thoughts and beliefs are helpful, or not. Without the qualities of slowing down, becoming still, and being silent, it is not always easy to access this level of reflective contemplation. Luckily, most people who come to restorative yoga find that they love it, and that the time slips away effortlessly. Unlike meditation, which at the start can be quite difficult and uncomfortable, restorative yoga makes it easy to relax, and so we are more likely to go back for more, and practise regularly.

Yoga nidra: lying down to wake up

Much like restorative yoga, yoga nidra also does not require any muscular strength or effort. It is a form of meditation practice, but more specifically, yoga nidra is a form of *guided meditation through relaxation*.

It takes us into a state of deep rest by deeply relaxing the body. We lie down, get warm and comfortable, and allow someone to guide us into a state of deep relaxation. Unlike restorative yoga which does require postural work with the body, albeit in a relaxed way, yoga nidra simply requires that you just lie down.

I still remember my first yoga nidra teacher training. I remember arriving home feeling like I was really glowing with happiness and peace. I saw the people getting on and off the trains bathed in radiant light, and nothing could have disturbed my sense of calm. It was a powerful experience, and one I am so grateful to have had, because in times of tension and stress, I recall that magical, peaceful feeling and I am reminded that everything—including today's tension and pain—is fleeting and transient. Change is made possible just by remembering times I have felt peaceful even if I don't have a practical or rational solution to my problems in that moment.

A (very) brief history

Yoga nidra is an old practice, and was brought to the attention of the West primarily by a yoga teacher named Satyananda. It was his style of teaching yoga nidra that influenced Dr Richard Miller, a doctor of clinical psychology, Sanskrit scholar, yoga teacher, and founder of iRest (which is an abbreviation for the Integrative Restoration Institute) based in North America, to develop yoga nidra to effectively reduce post-traumatic stress disorder (PTSD), depression, anxiety, insomnia, chronic pain, and chemical dependency while increasing health, resilience, and well-being. The third school of yoga nidra is from the Himalayan tradition, headed by yogi Swami Rama. For a practice reported to be over 2000 years old, it still carries great relevance for us today.

The structure and length of a yoga nidra meditation can vary depending on the style of yoga nidra being taught, but it is very common to be guided around each part of the body in the initial part of the sequence. This technique, sometimes called rotation of consciousness, helps the physical body begin to let go of tension. From being guided around the body, we may be invited to notice our breath, or to direct the breath around the body, for example, picturing the breath travelling evenly up one nostril to the eyebrow centre on the inhale, and then back down the other nostril on the exhale. We may be guided into visualisations, or we may experience periods of silence in the yoga nidra. A practice can be as little as ten minutes, as much as forty-five, and anyone can practise yoga nidra regardless of age, ability, or gender. As well as working with pairs of opposites, yoga nidra can involve body sensation, breath awareness, visualisation, sound, and working with the breath. It gives us the opportunity to experience moments of tranquillity and peace which can be enough to make us a yoga nidra devotee for life!

Waking sleep

Increasing studies are showing the positive changes that both yoga and meditation can have on the brain, including how yoga changes the brain wave patterns. Yoga nidra also brings about these positive changes, including activating the alpha and theta brain waves associated with mindfulness and imagination; but rather uniquely, unlike a more physical form of yoga practice, yoga nidra also activates the delta brain waves, the place of deep sleep, where healing and replenishment take place, with the beauty being that we don't need eight to ten hours sleep to get there. This is the reason that yoga nidra is so restful for the body, and such a tonic for worn out bodies, hearts, and souls.

The word nidra is Sanskrit, and often translated as meaning sleep, but I prefer Dr Richard Miller's translation, which is one of changing states of consciousness, as this seems more reflective of the fluid experience of yoga nidra. Much as when we sleep we go through stages of wakefulness, dreaming, and deep "dead to the world" sleep, we can go through this cycle in a twenty or thirty minute yoga nidra practice. We are never just asleep, but we are creating and dreaming and resting. Deep sleep has been described by Dr Matthew Edlund as "almost a state of consciousness yet is so close to coma you will not remember any of it."[1] Edlund is describing sleep, but this sounds to me very similar to yoga nidra. Yoga nidra is a journey to an awareness and presence that lies within us all. It is meditation through deep relaxation, and is wonderfully, beautifully a way of connecting back to your essence.

The recipe for Radical Rest

The tools of Radical Rest calm and relax us, our bodies, breath, minds, and hearts. We drop into being and we find the pleasure in simply being alive without needing anything more to be complete. To admire the morning skies and observe the change in temperature and light as seasons shift opens us up to a wonder that was always there. There is pleasure where perhaps there has only been pain, there is feeling where we have always felt numb, and we start to see the natural beauty and small acts of kindness, as well as acknowledging the mass consumption of potential terror and disaster we are fed.

We come back to life, better able to enjoy that home-cooked meal, the walk in the woods, or the time spent with friends and family. When we start to truly relax, our thoughts become lighter, our breath freer, and our body softer. We awaken more to creativity and find that we become more calm and steady, and so if something does happen in our life to scare or alarm us, we are able to be more responsive rather than reactive. This doesn't mean we are no longer scared, angry, aggressive, or ashamed—rather, we can open to the whole spectrum of our experience here without shutting up or rejecting parts of ourselves.

I remember a time when I had just moved house. It had been a big move for me, and I was feeling emotionally and physically unsettled. We were in the middle of a hot summer, but on this particular day it was pouring with rain, and I was inside, resting. There was a noise, and I went from the bedroom to the kitchen to find a man inside, with a dog, and a half drunk glass of beer in his hand. I was shocked, and asked if I could help him. My first reaction was that he had walked into the wrong flat, but the beer in his hand had me on high alert. It became clear that he didn't want to leave, and in fact seemed quite indignant that I should even ask him to go. At this time I had a whole range of thoughts running through my head—from my fears that he really wouldn't leave, to my irrational thoughts that I was being rude to ask him to go!—but when he looked at me and asked somewhat accusingly if I was a Christian, I firmly walked past him, opened the door, and told him he had to leave. He left, begrudgingly, and I phoned my husband who phoned the police. I share this story because I believe it was my regular yoga practice that helped me remain calm and in control of what could have been a much more terrifying experience.

Choose rest

When we first decide to make the choice to rest, rather than to be caught up in action, it can send ripples through our lives, and the more stressed, busy, and burnt out you are the bigger the ripples can be. And for me, as someone who had not rested in years (although admittedly had always slept well due to the sheer amount of activity I had crammed into each day), those ripples were more like waves, which washed over my entire being, and taught me, slowly and patiently, just how essential it was that I rested.

Starting any new activity can be difficult, and often takes some discipline and effort at the beginning. Luckily, the relaxing qualities of restorative yoga and yoga nidra are such that we find ourselves looking forward to our next session. We are so used to having to force ourselves into new health kicks and regimes that it can be quite startling to find ourselves drawn to something which we actually want to do! When we realise that what we really truly need is to rest more, and we are able to respond to that need, rather than resorting to old habits such as reaching for the extra coffee or just pushing ourselves extra hard, we are creating new actions and new thought patterns that can influence the rest of our day, and with regular practice, the rest of our lives.

It is by cultivating our awareness and understanding of ourselves that we really begin to know ourselves, and become clear about why we may be making the decisions and choices that we make. In my own case, by beginning to choose to rest (instead of waiting until I was exhausted or ill with no choice but to rest) I was choosing to accept myself, take care of myself, and respect myself, rather than put myself at the bottom of a list of importance. This, over time, changed my life, and perhaps it could change yours as well.

CHAPTER FIVE

You have been called to rest

Restless (adjective):
finding or affording no rest; uneasy, agitated; constantly in motion

Once upon a time I worked full time in marketing, communications, and fundraising in the charity sector. We used an expression, "call to action," as a way of making sure that each email or letter that we sent supporters had a clear action for that supporter to take. I came up with "call to rest" when I saw that this was what Radical Rest really was—a call from our bodies and minds to rest, to respond to the deep longing we feel down in our bones when we are worn out, and to remember our soulfulness, our essence as human beings, and in doing so alleviate the guilt that comes from needing rest.

Modern science has little time for abstract ideas of the soul, so you can interchange the word soul for psyche, or consciousness, if you feel more comfortable with that. However, many cultures, languages, religions, and schools of thought have had the notion of the soul for aeons, within religion, philosophy, and also within language.

In Greek the word *psyche pneuma* referred to breath and soul, and in Latin *anima spiritus* meant the same thing. In Japanese the word *ki* means air/spirit, and in Sanskrit, the ancient language of India and thus, yoga, the word *prana* refers to our life force, our vitality, which is expressed on the breath (the yogic practice of *pranayama* literally means extension of the life force).[1] We can see how breath and consciousness have been intricately linked for some time, and we will go on to explore the role of breath in stress, anxiety and the other Calls to Rest I go on to discuss.

Remembering who you really are ...

A Call to Rest is therefore a call from the soul to remember who we really are, beyond the lists and projects. It is the song of our hearts reminding us to look up and see the beauty around us, even in seemingly ordinary and mundane places and situations. Calls to Rest are symptoms of a restless society and exhausted individuals, and in the following chapters I look at stress, depression, anxiety, addiction, grief, trauma, and menstrual health problems as not only symptoms but messengers which are actually trying to help us.

This might sound peculiar, but if you recall the earlier chapter exploring the role of yoga and the mind-body connection, you will remember that the problems we experience in our body are often deeply related to the thoughts and beliefs that we carry in our mind. Although it is not easy to view something as debilitating as anxiety as a messenger, I will gently share practices of Radical Rest which can support you in learning to find your inner strength and resilience in the face of anxiety, depression, and more.

Whilst I have separated out these conditions, in spiritual teachings we learn that everything is connected. We also know that our experience is often multilayered, complex, and cannot be broken down into separate pieces. Depression often comes hand in hand with anxiety, trauma can lead to depression, addiction can come from anxiety and lead to depression, and trauma can result in addictions. Our disconnection with the Earth and our bodies can lead to a disconnection with our natural cycles, particularly the menstrual cycle.

Despite knowing the inaccuracy in dividing these topics into separate categories, I have nevertheless chosen to make each Call to Rest an individual chapter as it perhaps is easier for most of us to learn when information is laid out in a linear fashion. I certainly found researching the topics easier when I divided them from one another, but as my research deepened over time and my contemplation of what I was finding developed, it suddenly felt somewhat inept to be talking about these subjects as though they were in no way related to each other. However, the chapters are still presented in this way for ease of understanding.

All the calls to rest I deal with are experiences which can feel so isolating and yet are so common. This is not an exhaustive list, but these are areas with which I have had personal experience, and so I write from the viewpoint of my work with clients, my own practice, and personal experience as a human being who still stumbles from time to time. Each of the following chapters suggests a restorative yoga posture which may help with that particular issue. Remember that restorative yoga is designed to be effortless and restful, but if in doubt, check with a qualified teacher. Although I suggest a particular posture, I also will cross-reference postures from other chapters. I invite you to explore all the postures and see what works for you. Your preferences and experiences may change each time you do the practice, even if these changes are subtle. Trust your instincts. I have done my best to make the instructions clear and concise, but if you are not sure, contact your local restorative yoga teacher and seek his or her opinion.

Each chapter contains a breathing practice to bring calm and balance to the mind. As I mentioned before, breathing practices in yoga are called "pranayama," the extension of our life force, with the idea being that any time we are focusing our mental energy towards our breath we are connecting deeply with our life force, that which sustains us and keeps us here. Physiologically speaking, when we are stressed, worried, or feeling out of balance, our breath may become shallow, frozen, short, or quick. By practising restorative yoga postures first of all you will relax muscular tension which will free up your breath. This will make the breathing exercises easier. Once you have got into a regular habit of practising Radical Rest, you may find you can go straight to the breathing exercises, although it's important to note that if you feel stressed or tense while doing the breathing exercises then you should stop immediately and practise the restorative yoga posture instead.

Finally, each section ends with a link to obtain a free yoga nidra recording, designed to help you to completely let go. These are my personal favourite Radical Rest tools, forms of conscious action which takes us into a state of deep rest, and following the Calls to Rest I will explore in a philosophical and soulful way how we got to be in a state where stress, anxiety, and depression were all so commonplace, and why there is always light at the end of the tunnel, always.

You may like to read through all Calls to Rest, or there may be one which really does "call" to you. However you chose to explore the next few chapters, be patient and give yourself time to reflect upon the ideas mentioned. Some may be new, some of the concepts may be difficult to get your head around, but remember that this is a look at health problems from a soulful perspective. That is not to say I disagree with medical or other more orthodox viewpoints, on the contrary I support wholeheartedly a rounded and intelligent discussion on the subject of well-being, but my experiences and most likely my personality have led me to reflect more philosophically than scientifically, towards the more abstract than logical. I have included some of my research from people far more expert in these fields than me, but mainly my observations come from my years of practice, of teaching, of study, and of reflection. The topics I have selected are incredibly weighty, and are worthy of books of their own, and I have recommended some books I have found to be very useful at the back of this book.

As you read, remember principles two and four—be curious yet cautious. Take time to reflect on the points I make, and decide how you think and feel about them. Try the practices, and see the impact they have on you. This is not about my way being the right way but one of the many ways of reflecting on the self. Radical Rest most certainly is not a panacea, but I hope it can offer you perhaps a new way of dealing with some of the issues so many of us are tackling in everyday life. We humans are deeply interconnected beings, affected by the way we work, communicate, think, and feel as much as we are influenced by genetics and hormones, so I don't believe anything out there could work for everybody. Enjoy, discuss, and share your reflections—and don't forget to practise. Yoga is embodied philosophy and it is never fully experienced until we put the theory into practice, the philosophy into activity.

A final note, our bodies are made to move. If you are currently undertaking any other physical activity which you are confident is replenishing your energy and not depleting it, then you do not need to give it up in order to practise Radical Rest. Radical Rest can complement a healthy active lifestyle, as well as nourish those of us who are exhausted. I practised daily for about five years. I was deeply exhausted, living on stress, anxiety, and constant activity. Yoga nidra was at first a tonic providing deep rest; now it is mostly a meditation practice (although I will often use it as a way to rest deeply when I'm feeling tired). I of course do still get tired, do still fall into the trap of overdoing, but I am much more responsive when this happens. I work much more with my menstrual cycle and the seasons, and have developed a greater respect for my body and my needs to rest. The amount you need to practise will be up to you, but certainly a daily practice can be hugely transformative. Never under-estimate the beauty and peace that comes from daily relaxation.

A note on purchasing equipment

Most yoga equipment is relatively inexpensive, with the exception of bolsters (long firm cushions designed to provide support and comfort). If you plan to practise restorative yoga regularly it's worth investing in a bolster, but at the beginning you can substitute some firm pillows for bolsters. Remember you want to feel relaxed and comfortable in a posture: if you're not sure you are doing it right, consult a qualified restorative yoga teacher (your local yoga studio or gym should be able to offer advice).

A yoga mat is essential and these range widely in price. It's worth getting something with some grip (especially if you plan to use the mat for more vigorous types of yoga), but you certainly don't have to get the most expensive one you can find. Yoga straps (sometimes referred to as belts) and eye pillows (like bean bags, often lightly scented with lavender), are relatively inexpensive and easy to buy online. If you feel inclined, why not make your own? There are articles online about how to do this. You may choose to invest to buy yoga blocks and bricks, but again don't feel as though you have to purchase loads of pricey equip-ment in order to practise restorative yoga; it's amazing what you can do with cushions, pillows, and old scarves!

Two of the postures involve the use of a yoga chair. These are bespoke items and you may not be willing to invest in such a thing. However, they are one of my personal favourite pieces of restorative yoga kit. You can replicate some of the postures by stacking up bolsters and cushions or using your sofa, bed or footstool, but it is important that these feel stable and not as though they are about to fall over at any moment. If you are unable to successfully replace the use of a chair and do not want to pur-chase a chair, then simply try one of the other postures that I recommend.

Sometimes a timer is useful. If you have one on your phone feel free to use it, but remember to put your phone onto flight mode first, to avoid any distractions during your practice. The breathing practices work well after restorative yoga, but can be done on their own once you feel relaxed and at ease with them. Yoga nidra can be done at any time in isolation or in conjunction with any of the other Radical Rest tools.

Getting ready to practise Radical Rest

Restorative yoga is more of a softening than a stretching. Each posture should be fairly comfortable, although if you are brand new to yoga be aware than sometimes the postures may feel unusual. Certainly there should never be any pain. Because the postures are more passive than active, you should be able to go straight into them. However, I have included a few more active preparatory stretches that you might like to do before going into the restorative yoga postures.

Preparation stretches

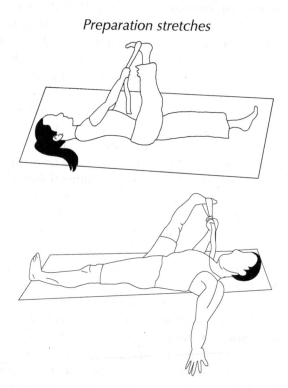

Hamstring stretch (in Sanskrit, supta padangusthasana A & B).

What you need:

It is useful to have a yoga strap for this stretch, although an old scarf may suffice. You need something that you can press your foot into securely.

How to do it:

- Start by lying on your back on a firm but warm surface, knees bent. Place a soft cushion or folded blanket under your head.
- Starting on the right side, bring your right knee in towards your chest, and place the strap over the ball of the foot (just beneath the toes).
- As you inhale, straighten your leg as much as is comfortable as though you were going to stand on the ceiling. Your left leg stays bent, or if you are comfortable you can straighten it (as in the illustration).
- Hold the strap in both hands to keep space for the shoulders. Relax the neck and jaw. Breathe deep into your belly. As you exhale, relax the shoulders towards the floor. Press your foot up towards the ceiling as you keep releasing your buttock towards the floor. Stay for 1–2 minutes then prepare for the second stage.
- The next stage requires support next to the hips. If you have yoga equipment you can use a block and a brick, otherwise cushions are fine. Now hold both ends of the strap with your right hand. Place your left arm on the floor beside you in line with your shoulder with the palm facing up. If you straightened your left leg, bend it again. Keeping the right leg straight and the left knee bent, let the legs move let the legs move away from one another keeping the belly button and the gaze pointing up to the ceiling. Your blocks or cushions should provide support for the hips as they open. Stay here for 1–2 minutes breathing fully.
- To come out, breathe in deeply and bring the legs back towards one another. As you exhale, bend the right knee in to the chest, release the strap, and place the foot on the floor. Both legs should be bent, feet on the floor.
- Repeat on the other side.

Useful for:

This is a wonderful way to prepare for the posture I have called Receiving Posture, also known as supta baddha konasana or reclined bound angle pose. This is the posture recommended in the section on menstrual health, because it stretches the inner thighs and prepares the hips to open. It can also be useful to do this before the legs up wall posture explored in the chapter on grief. It's also very helpful for anyone who runs, walks, cycles, or sits in a chair for long periods of times as it helps to stretch the hamstrings and release tension in the lower back.

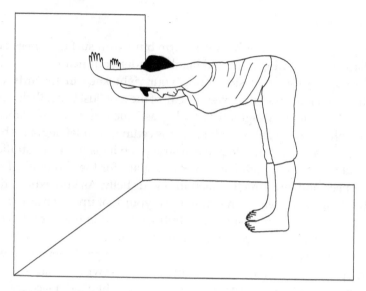

Down Dog at wall (in Sanskrit, adho mukha svanasana).

What you need:

A wall

How to do it:

- Stand facing the wall. Be barefooted to avoid the risk of slipping, and use a yoga mat.
- Place your hands against the wall in line with the shoulders, placing them slightly wider than shoulder width apart.
- Begin to walk the feet backwards as you walk the hands down the wall.
- Do not take your hands lower than shoulder height. At most, your torso will be parallel with the floor, but you do not need to go to this extreme to feel the benefit of the stretch.
- Once in position begin to press the hands firmly into the wall while bending your knees softly and pressing your heels down.
- You can deepen the stretch in the back of the body by pressing your hips back and straightening the legs. Do not straighten your legs if your hamstrings are tight or lower back is sore.
- Stay for 1–2 minutes, breathing deeply.

- When you are ready to come out, inhale, and begin to walk the feet back towards the wall. Walk your hands up the wall, and keep them on the wall until you are upright. If you feel dizzy you may have gone too low in the posture, or walked out of the posture too quickly. In this case, rest your hands on top of one another on the wall, and rest your forehead on your arms for a few breaths until the dizziness has passed.

Useful for:

This is a useful way to stretch the whole back of the body and can be done at any time of day. It may be particularly useful as a way to prepare for child's pose, given in the section on anxiety, or the downward twist in the chapter on addiction.

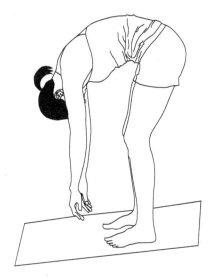

Spinal roll.

What you need:

Nothing, just a floor to stand on!

How to do it:

- Stand with the feet hip distance apart.
- Have a soft bend in the knees, and begin to let the head curl down towards the chest.

- Keep the knees lightly bent as you continue to curl forward. The intention is not to get the hands to the floor but to deeply stretch the back of the body.
- Let the arms hang heavily.
- You may like to gently rock from side to side here, keeping the arms dangling heavily, or if you prefer, holding each elbow with the opposing hand.
- You can also take a gentle twist to each side while hanging over the legs. Make sure you turn from the hips, not the knees. The knees should stay pointing forward the whole time.
- To come out of the posture press down firmly with the soles of the feet, keep the knees softly bent, and as you inhale slowly come back up to standing. Head is the last to lift.

Useful for:

This is a wonderful morning stretch, and useful to do if you are spending hours at your desk. You can do it in preparation for any of the postures I suggest in the subsequent chapters, but it may be particularly useful for the downward twist given in the section of addiction.

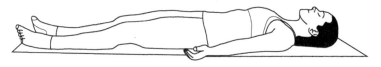

Posture: Savasana, or lying down relaxation posture.

What you need:

Just a surface to lie on. This can be your bed (although bear in mind that you may fall asleep), or on the floor.

How to do it:

Nice and simple, this involves simply resting onto your back. You may like to use an eye pillow for extra relaxation, particularly if you feel that you have been mentally active for most of the day. You may like to place a cushion or bolster under the backs of the knees to help the lower back to settle.

Useful for:

Completely resting the body, reducing any muscular effort, and letting go of the need to be "doing."

Many thanks go to yoga teacher Donna Farhi, who inspired some of these postures. More details of these, and many others, can be found in her book, *The Breathing Book.*

Note on breathing exercises:

Each of the breathing exercises offers a description of how to do it, why it works, alternative practices to try, and importantly, what to watch out for. The breath is a very powerful tool that is both under our conscious and unconscious control. This means that we don't need to think about it in order to do it—which is lucky, considering it keeps us alive—but that we *can* think about and change it, if we want. When the body is stressed and tense, it is not really worth trying to change the breath in any way. Instead it is more effective to relax the body and create space for the breath. All the breathing practices can be done in isolation, but when you are new to yoga, it can be easier to start with the restorative yoga practices, then when you feel ready, move onto the breathing exercise. When in doubt, please ask the advice of an experienced yoga teacher. It can be enough to work just with the body for some time before you feel ready to work with the breath. Particularly if there is any high blood pressure, epilepsy, or heart condition, please seek the advice of your medical professional before beginning. The breath should never be held during pregnancy.

CHAPTER SIX

Call to rest: Stress

Stress, the malady of the modern world. We say we're stressed so often that it no longer comes as a surprise to us or those around us. We have accepted stress as a part of life to manage, and whilst on the one hand that is completely accurate, on the other hand stress has moved beyond the status of a physiological response to a frightening situation, and become somewhat of a badge of honour, a status symbol even, and a sign of a successful modern life.

I remember a friend of mine working under stressful conditions for an accountancy firm. He was racking up continuous late nights at the office trying to meet tight deadlines when his manager called him in. She accused him of "not caring enough" about the work. Her reason for thinking this? He wasn't panicking, he wasn't creating a big drama and making sure everyone knew how hard he was working but he was *quietly* working as hard as he could to get things done. Yet in the competitive workplace it wasn't enough to just get work done, you had to be *seen* as being incredibly stressed to prove how hard you were working.

Thriving or surviving?

Despite how many of us describe ourselves as feeling stressed, stress itself is a personal and felt experience. What stresses me out might may seem like a minor thing to you, whereas what causes you stress might be highly motivating to someone else. I might experience stress by fighting it, trying to control it and in doing so attempting to control myself, from my diet to my exercise regime. Other people may pull back from life and lose any sense of what they think or feel about things, preferring to go along with the crowd and lose their autonomy.[1] Saying we're stressed then doesn't always tell us an awful lot about what we're actually experiencing when under too much pressure, but the reasons we are stressed can and do vary from person to person. Certainly it's important to remember that stress is not just a feeling in your head, but something which causes the whole body to react accordingly.

We've all probably heard the story of the caveman encountering a tiger. In that moment the ever-so-clever brain recognises danger and the fight or flight response is activated. The heart rate increases, breath becomes shallow and rapid, and the muscles tense up, so the caveman can run away from the tiger, or less likely, try to fight it, hence fight or flight. Many of us don't have this problem to contend with (there's definitely not too many tigers where I live) but we do have phantom tigers, like managing our finances, creating careers, and balancing all the demands of life which are stressing us out.

None of these phantom tigers are going to kill us on the spot, but neither can we run away from them. We don't need our heart rate to increase, our breath to quicken, or our muscles to tense so we can pay our bills on time but when our situation makes us stressed, our brains activate a fight or flight response, regardless of the cause. We can't "fight or flight" our way out of the responsibility of monthly payments, and those worries about the future may never go away, and so in these instances fight or flight isn't really that helpful, but that doesn't stop the brain responding in the same way as if a tiger were looking at us and licking his lips.

When we feel constantly under threat, we get worn down. Things that we may have taken in our stride a few months earlier suddenly send us into a state of panic and tension, we may find our digestion is not what it was, our sleep deteriorates, and our desire for sex completely disappears. Stress also affects our metabolism, our growth, our ability to conceive, our ability to feel pain, our memory, our mental health, and our ability to enjoy life. And get this, even with extreme wealth and power we may still be operating in survival mode.

How can this be? Surely we've been taught that wealth and power is the end goal, that this is what brings satisfaction and success, but as we know these things are fleeting and in the capitalist society we live in, there will always be someone richer and someone more powerful than you, and even they may be caught in fight or flight. Is there a solution to managing stress? Consider this idea for a moment: when we say we are stressed, we are really saying we are afraid. Fight or flight is a physiological response to a situation when we feel under threat, aka, when we are fearful.

If stress is fear, then our biggest fear is often death, loss, and pain. The worries of daily survival may take up most of our energy, but beneath the bills and the workload is a fear of loss. The literal experience of dying is not something many of us care to think about, and for good reasons. Life matters to us, no matter how hard or trying it can seem and so it should: to embrace life, love life is a wonderful, wonderful thing. But we do live in a culture which values youth and beauty, vitality and extravagance and this makes dealing with death (which we all have to do at some point whether it is facing our own or experiencing the death of a loved one) something we are often completely ill-prepared for, and something money and power can't help us with.

The only thing we can do is to begin to develop our spiritual selves (which can go quite happily hand in hand with attaining money and power, if those things are used in a way to benefit all), and in doing so, begin to find an inner resource which supports us and nourishes us in our daily and often stressful life. When we work to overcome the ultimate fear of dying, we become free to deal with the "mini" stresses of money, work, and to-do lists.

Me, myself, and I

In the yoga tradition, as in other spiritual practices and also disciplines like psychotherapy, there is the concept of the ego. The ego is the part of us that labels the world around us, and comes up with our sense of self. It is who we call "I". It is the part of us that realises our own willpower and autonomy—think of a toddler throwing a tantrum as one fully expressing willpower!—but it is also the part of us that is scared of death, loss, and pain.

Traditionally yoga was used as a way to overcome the ego self and to merge completely with the Divine. It was thought that the ego distracted us from the peaceful state of meditation we would otherwise be in.[2] For dedicated yogis, prepared to give up "ordinary" life and spend years of solitude in meditation upon a mountain top, the ego indeed would be a distraction. It would remind you there was no chocolate to be found up there, and how much you used to enjoy the cinema, and thus distract you from your enlightenment (tongue firmly in cheek there).

For those of us not on that path (or indeed on that mountain top) we don't have to overcome the ego to practise yoga or manage our stresses and fears. The ego itself is not a bad thing but investing only in the ego is like buying a plant pot but forgetting to pot the plant. A healthy ego creates a healthy container for our radiant spiritual selves to emerge and grow out into the world, to do the work that we came here to do, to learn the lessons we must learn, and pass on the wisdom we gather. An unhealthy ego forgets all of that and keeps us feeling unsafe and highly stressed as it clings onto impermanent fleeting values like youth, beauty, wealth, and power. Sounds familiar? Those values are only sold to you in every advertisement you ever saw, every celebrity magazine you secretly browsed, and every beauty product you've bought.

Whilst a certain amount of income and autonomy is important for securing our physical needs and alleviating the basic stress of survival, we are often told that we need more, must work harder, earn more money, buy a house, then buy a bigger house. The drive for more and more material possessions and ownership easily becomes a trap and we forget the value of time spent with friends and family, time spent on hobbies we do just for the love of it, and the beauty in watching the rain fall or the sun rise.

The idea of failure and success are products of the ego. We may perceive that we have failed at something based on our own ideas of what success looks like or judge ourselves by society's idea of success, but when we move away from fixed and rigid definitions we might see our journeys through life as a series of lessons and experiences. Achieving only wealth and status becomes less important as our values begin to shift. I certainly found this when I first started teaching yoga—I was so delighted that people came to my classes and workshops that the work was a source of happiness to me. In my professional career I was so anxious to achieve more security through working more hours and earning more money that any success I had was paled by my need to have more. This was less to do with greed and more to do with my own fears. I had convinced myself that the only way to feel safe was to work hard, and it seemed that I could never work hard enough to feel safe.

It was my belief and attitude that drove me to work in a way that was stressful. Work can be, as I since realised, a joy. Exercise can be fun, eating healthily can be a pleasure, and living off less money can actually create more time as you realise you didn't need all the stuff you thought you did. In essence, when we understand our drive, our motivation, and start to heal ourselves at the source, the way we experience stress can change. Stress can be created from our perception of events as much as the events themselves. Stress can be created when we feel powerless or when we feel power-obsessed. Two people doing the same job may have a completely different experience of it.

Although stress is inevitable, when we start to recognise that we can cultivate healthy willpower, develop inner confidence, and rise to life's challenges then we can create a healthy and balanced ego that can meet the demands of the world while setting clear boundaries and developing spiritual awareness. Cool, huh? The stress of fear has to be met with the acknowledgement of our vulnerability. We must accept that one day we will die but that in the meantime we have a whole rich life to live. Unless we awaken to the potential in each moment then we continue to suffer from the stress created by fear. When we look beyond the stresses that can make us feel so alone, we start to recognise what unites us, what binds us, what holds us together as families, friends, lovers, workers, citizens, nations, and perhaps sooner than we know, earthlings.

It is crucial that we all start to look beyond the stories we've been told so far, because all around us we see the dismantling of the structures and belief systems that once defined us. Stories of abuse in both religious and spiritual institutions abound, divisive politics are vying for power in a political framework which is broken, and corruption rules. While the old structures and out of date ideologies come crumbling down, they aren't going down without a fight. Until we remember that we are reliant on the Earth to grow our food and give us clean water then we stay trapped in our belief that money and status can save us and that the price of chronic stress is one we are happy to carry in exchange for feeling safe. The future is uncertain and that scares us. Beginning to see life as a cycle (not a linear one-way A to B route) can help us manage life's disappointments, and our perceived failures, and we become stronger. We can use stress as a tool to understand ourselves, realise when we need to make changes, and grow rather than stagnate or feel defeated, as though we were born to live stressed-out, anxious lives, rather than lives full of love, laughter and joy.

Whether you think you can or you can't, you're right[3]

Although some aspects of stress may be beyond our control, we might also acknowledge to ourselves that we are creating some aspects of our stressful life for ourselves. If we are bored or unfulfilled in our work we may actually crave stress as a way to keep ourselves stimulated or motivated, or if we are simply tired, a rush of stress hormones might give us that boost to get through the day. A lack of money might cause us to overwork, unhappiness with our image might cause us to over-exercise, a fear of stillness might cause us to overdo, and when driven by fear, we create stress. This is different to working for the love of it, of exercising because we love our bodies and want them to feel good. This comes down to intention and understanding: why do we do what we do?

Remember that when we feel stressed we are not making a conscious choice to feel stressed. This isn't about blaming yourself for not being more resilient or capable, but realising that feeling stressed, activating fight or flight, may be something your brain is *defaulting* to as it tries to prepare you for the perceived or real dangers ahead. This is actually an intelligent response of the brain as it tries to protect us in the best way it knows how. It's just that this response can get old, and become ineffective as we grow and develop as people.

We can't always change our situation. We can't change what has happened to us in the past. But there is always something we can do in this moment whether that involves seeking help or accepting our situation as it is right now. Acceptance is different to resignation: when we accept we find we have the power to create space in our life for the changes we desire. Knowing our job is demanding and stressful and hating or resenting it is different from knowing our job is demanding and stressful yet accepting that that is how it is *in the present moment* and that the present moment is always changing. This brings a subtle shift in thought and energy. It can somehow lift the load, if we let it. And sometimes, surprisingly, we start to see ways out. Remember that this is hard to do when we feel stressed, but Radical Rest can help us relax enough to clear the mind and create space for change to take place.

As an aside, stress isn't always bad for us. There are always two sides to every coin, and this means that stress can even be good for us.

Stress can also help us to get a piece of important and meaningful work completed in time to meet a deadline, or cross the finish line of the race we've trained so fervently for. In these situations, stress could actually help us to prepare to meet some of the challenges we face. It might sound crazy, but learning to make friends with stress may be the first step in learning how to reduce stress and manage the unavoidable stress we all experience in life.

Making friends with stress doesn't mean you deny the stress that you're under. It certainly doesn't mean you give in to the pressure that you're under at work, especially if it's from bullying or unrealistic expectations of your role from others, but what it does mean is that you start to accept that there will be stress in life, and understand what you could do to better respond to it. This may begin with taking some time to reflect on what causes you stress in your life, and how much control you have over each situation. This is more easily achieved after a practice of Radical Rest rather than in the middle of a crisis! While we may not be able to do much about the traffic jam we're in, or about the colleague who sends emails at 11 at night and 7 in the morning, we can increase our self-awareness so that we can learn to recognise our own stress triggers, and develop strategies to deal with stress. Warning: stress can be addictive. The ability to check email and social media at any time of day, the ability to stay late and arrive early in the office, and the ability to survive (for a while, at least) on takeaway coffee and "convenience" food makes it easier for us to feed the addictive habits that cause us stress. More on addiction in Chapter 8.

Love is the answer, no matter what the question

One of the hormones released when we are stressed is oxytocin, the hormone that encourages us to seek help, to look for compassion and human connection, according to psychologist Kelly McGonigal.[4] I love this idea, because as someone who hasn't always been comfortable with asking for help, preferring instead to struggle on alone, the realisation that my stressed-out body was trying to encourage me to listen to my heart reassures me that it's OK to ask for help. It's OK to feel tired and yes, occasionally stressed out. I am reminded again of the mind-body connection and the innate wisdom of our bodies. Not only can stress encourage us to ask for help, but it also acts as a warning sign, telling us that we may need to pay more attention to the actions we are taking and the thoughts and beliefs driving them.

In a culture where our world leaders are criticised if they show human emotion and where failure is often not an option, vulnerability doesn't score too highly on the list of sought-after emotions. Being vulnerable very often is associated with being weak, scared, or at higher risk to threat, and while no one wants (or needs) to feel vulnerable all the time, accessing our vulnerability can help us to recognise our need for help and support.

The power of you

There is power in asking for help and we have more power than we realise. Most of us do have a certain amount of say in how we spend the whole day be that what time we wake up to how we spend our lunch break, what food we eat, and what we do after work. While some of life's stresses are inevitable, some of them we create all on our own, yet so many of us are unaware or too afraid to acknowledge our power and instead fall into the trap of seeing constant productivity and action as secrets to success. When our actions are not led from the heart, when our productivity is to someone else's gain, we can experience stress, and over time, its good friend burnout.

When we lose ourselves in our pursuit for someone else's idea of success, be that in the workplace or at the gym, then we lose the connection with our body that tells us when to pull back, to do less, and rest more. We get caught in a cycle of doing-doing-doing until the day we literally can't get out of bed in the morning. This might sound extreme, but is more common than you may realise, and not just with jet-setting celebrities. As well as the physical implications, burnout can make us more negative, cynical, and less productive at work, yet how many of us have gambled with our health and well-being by staying late in the office or "just checking my emails" before bed?

Taking back some control over our lives can sound impossible, unrealistic, or just plain terrifying to most of us. We may blame ourselves for getting burnt out, for not dealing with stress better, and in doing so create a self-perpetuating cycle of blame and shame, neither of which ever led to empowerment. When you realise how strong you really are, and you redefine strength as being authentic in your vulnerability, you create a sense of presence in yourself that elevates you from the very real stresses of survival, and gives you access to the spiritual dimension of life.

How Radical Rest helps

Radical Rest can help us recover from stress and burnout by giving us the chance to rest deeply and start to heal. Over time we create new stories, new thoughts, and new possibilities that can create a new future for ourselves. It may seem like a small step for some, but the actions you take every day are creating your life, and the power of your imagination is extraordinary.

Imagining a stressful situation can cause our body to respond in exactly the same way as if that stressful situation were to happen, that's how clever our brains are. This means that by worrying about all the things that could go wrong, or finding ourselves stuck in a cycle of negative thought patterns and rumination, we may be triggering the stress response when everything on the outside is actually OK. That is how powerful our thoughts are: they shape our world and experience, but regardless of whether our stress is real, perceived, or imagined, it would appear that for many of us, stress is no longer a fleeting sensation, a rare and extreme experience which our fight or flight response is built to handle, but instead has become a constant state of being. Imagine if that state of being was one of relaxation and rest, with stress being the momentary visitor? It is possible when we practise relaxation every day, but be warned: when we first let ourselves rest, we may actually feel worse.

Exhaustion might truly hit us, we become aware of the well of emotion within us, we feel listless and lost, and of course, we can feel vulnerable, and perhaps this is why so many of us avoid it, like I did for many years. When we drop away all the tasks and goals that define us, we can feel empty. This is part of letting go of the ego, but if we're wrapped up in the ego self then it can feel terrible. It certainly wasn't easy for me! I had wrapped so much of myself in my work that when I started to let it go it was incredibly hard. Radical Rest helped me then, and it can help you to explore stillness and "non-doing," to step away from the ego and get comfortable with a sense of nothingness.

After time we find it not only becomes easier to be with those quiet points in life but we actually crave it. As much as we are sold the idea of yoga challenges and expensive green powders as tools of well-being, to find out what we really desire in this life requires slowing down, stillness, and perhaps a bit of solitude in order to contemplate on our values and desires. Without rest we have no clarity and without clarity we have no insight. Without insight we lack the imagination to create a better future for ourselves and the world, and as that legend Maxi Jazz once said, you don't need eyes to see, you need vision.

With scaremongering and confusion in our media around climate change, politics, and so-called fake news, we need more than facts and rational analysis to find solutions: we need bright sparks, bright ideas, and ambition. And when was the last time you had any of those in a sleep-deprived, stressed-out moment? Too much rushing around, trying to be all things to all people, merely takes us further away from ourselves, leaving us confused about what we want to be and becoming watered down versions of who we could be. This is where Radical Rest comes in, as a tool to take us out of fight or flight and a method to guide us back into a more balanced and restful state of being.

Humans are creative, adaptable, and beautiful beings. We are so often shown the shadow qualities of humans, the pain and suffering that is caused, that we forget to see the power held within the daily shows of love and kindness shared between strangers holding the door for one another, between a parent setting their child off to school. Life brings its ups and downs, no one can escape that and nor should we want to. It is through our learning of life's lessons, the deepening of our experiences that we truly find a sense of who we are, and that self is rooted not in our job title, not in our bank balance, not even in our physical body, but is rooted in our acknowledgement of ourselves as beings who are human, imperfect, and messy, but Divine all the same. The more we answer the call from stress to listen to our hearts, the more we manage the stress that comes our way and the more we find deeper down what we need right now.

Ultimately it is our love for ourselves and our fellow creatures that can alleviate the feelings of daily stress. The more we let ourselves rest, the more we relax into the wonder and beauty of the day. On the other hand, the more time we spend in a state of chronic stress, the longer the stress hormones stay in our bodies, maybe for a prolonged period of time. Even if we think we're relaxing now we're home from work, our body might still be in a state of stress, and just like needing that first cup of coffee, we are at risk of craving more stimulation, more distraction. It's why it's so important that we can take time to relax every day, remove the day's tensions, and start afresh the next day. Making a conscious choice to relax (and Radical Rest is of course one way, but not the only way, to do this) helps you become an active participant in your own life, rather than a passive receiver in the unfolding of events around you.

Radical Rest

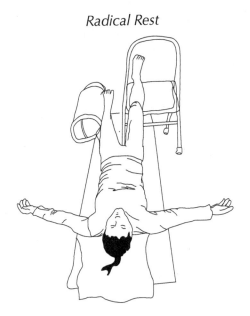

Restorative yoga posture: relaxation on chair.

What you need:

You will need something of suitable height that you can rest the backs of your calves comfortably on. I use a yoga chair, but you can also experiment by piling up bolsters and cushions or using a footstool, your sofa or bed. If you do use a chair of some sort, make sure it has a warm and soft padding on the seats. You will also need blankets to lie on, a blanket or cushion for the head, and perhaps a blanket to keep you warm. It can also be helpful to place a bolster or cushion next to the ankle of the leg that is not on the chair seat to stop the ankle from flopping out to the side. Like all the postures, you may like to use an eye pillow.

How to do it:

Make sure you have a comfortable and warm surface to lie on. A blanket folded over the top of a yoga mat works well. If you do use a chair of some sort, make sure at least two of its feet are on the sticky mat, or some sort of a surface where it will not slip. Make sure it has a warm and soft padding on the seats. Yoga chairs are made of metal and so I usually fold a blanket on the chair seat. Sit facing the chair, and then shift the chair over a few degrees to the right side. Make sure you have a bolster or firm cushion nearby to the left side of the chair. Place your right leg onto the chair seat, making sure the back of the knee touches the edge of the chair seat. Carefully lower yourself down onto your back, using your elbows and arms for support. Allow space for your left leg to comfortably straighten so it is next to the chair (not under). Once you are lying comfortably on your back, straighten the left leg and adjust the bolster so that it is resting next to the left ankle (you may need someone to assist you with this). Your left ankle should be in line with your left hip. Cover your chest with a blanket. You can relax here for up to twenty minutes on each side. When you are ready to come out, bend your left leg, bring your right knee towards your chest and roll carefully to one side. Rest on your side of a few breaths, before using your arms to push yourself up to sitting. Repeat on the other side, remembering to shift the chair off-centre, in the direction to the left.

Why it works:

Oh my word, is this posture good. I have never seen anything else work so efficiently when it comes to bringing instant peace to a room of students. This posture calms and soothes the nervous system almost straight away. It helps to soften and lengthen the psoas muscle, a deep hip flexor that helps the leg move forward and backward (think walking). When we're under a lot of stress, this muscle can get tight and dry. The impact of this is that the breathing becomes shorter and more shallow, which can exacerbate feelings of stress and anxiety. Try not to rush around after you've completed the posture. Instead just walk around a little, let the legs swing and the feet really land on the floor. I have to thank the London based yoga teacher Anna Ashby for sharing this posture with me: it's just so good.

Watch out for:

This posture is safe for everyone, unless you are pregnant and uncomfortable lying flat on your back. Certainly women in the third trimester should not lie on their backs, but women in earlier stages of pregnancy may also find lying on the back uncomfortable. For women in this stage of pregnancy, I recommend the restorative yoga posture shared in Chapter 12 on menstrual health as an alternative to this posture. You might like to have lots of blankets so you can place one on the chair (particularly if you're using a metal chair), as well as to lie on, and a blanket folded under the head. If there is any injury around the inner groin, be careful as you straighten the leg that is not on the chair. This posture should help, but always move slowly, and listen to your body.

Also try:

If this posture doesn't work for you, or you don't have anything suitable on which to prop up your leg, try the Effortless Rest posture on page 122. All of the postures suggested in this book provide excellent stress relief, so you really can explore what helps you feel more relaxed and calm. If you are heavily pregnant, and/or in the third trimester, avoid all postures which involve lying flat on your back. Instead, try the posture given in the chapter on menstrual health (page 138).

Stress breathing exercise: balancing breath

How to do it:

Start by noticing your breath in its current state. Notice if it is fast, slow, steady, erratic. When you feel ready to begin, sit comfortably. Try to maintain a long spine. Lift your right arm, and place your right thumb lightly against the nostril, at the soft fleshy bit. Your index finger should be able to reach the same side of the left nostril. When you are ready to begin, gently close the left nostril and breathe in through the right nostril. Breathe out through the right nostril, keeping gentle pressure on the left nostril. That is one breath. Repeat 5 times on the right side, then switch to the left, and repeat again 5 times. Repeat on both nostrils so that you have taken 25 breaths through each nostril. You may like to sit quietly for a few moments after, or if you feel tired, lie down and rest.

Why it works:

This breath aims to bring a sense of balance back to the system. Particularly when the mind is racing or distracted, after a few rounds of this exercise, the mind can become quieter and more still. This is a version of nadi shodhana, the yoga breathing exercise meaning "purify the flow," also known as alternate nostril breath.

Watch out for:

With all breathing practices, stop immediately if you feel stressed, anxious, or unwell. Most of us have spent our whole lives not thinking about our breath. To try to force the breath in any way is unproductive. Instead think of this as an invitation to change the flow and direction of the breath. Be curious, and explore what happens. Don't worry if you can't concentrate at the beginning and you keep losing count. With practice, it will become easier.

Also try:

You may like to explore all the practices suggested throughout the book to help you reduce stress in the body. The lion's roar as described on page 83 in Chapter 8 on addiction can be a way to bring some light-hearted fun into your day. The practice in Chapter 10 on grief can be a helpful way to create some space in the body if you have been rushing around and perhaps taking short, rapid, or shallow breaths, or perhaps even holding the breath.

Yoga nidra for stress:

This yoga nidra is designed to help relax the whole physical body, and awaken a sense of freshness and creativity within us. Access this recording for free via my website www.melskinneryoga.com/free-yoga-nidra and use the password RestIsRadical!

CHAPTER SEVEN

Call to rest: Anxiety

It's hard to talk about stress and fear then *not* lead straight onto anxiety in the next breath. They go hand in hand. The crisis and disaster fed to us in every news bulletin creates feelings of fear and worry about situations we can usually do little, if anything, about. Add to this our fears over our individual health, happiness, and personal safety, our worries for our loved ones, and our concerns for the future and we can start to feel as though we're stuck on high alert, just waiting for the apocalypse.

Anxiety, like stress, has its roots in the body. Science studies this through psychology, immunology, and neuroscience known collectively as psychoneuroimmunology. There is even the science of psychoneuro-immunoendocrinology, if you really want to win at Scrabble (although good luck trying to find a Scrabble board big enough to fit this word on!). This mouthful of a word which includes the role of the hormonal system is, according to Dr Gabor Maté, "the unity of emotions and physiology in human development and through life in health and illness."[1]

This is in essence the mind-body connection. Anxiety can be experienced as shortness of breath, as our inability to relax fully in the present moment for fear of what may happen prevents us from breathing fully and deeply. The mind starts to race. We may feel dizzy, unsteady on our feet, as though the whole world is spinning in front of us, the heart may beat faster, the body may begin to ache, and while classified as a mental health condition, it most certainly is not just in our head. Our whole body participates in the experience and anyone who has experienced anxiety knows that it can be debilitating. It is not something to be underestimated or lightly written off, but something that can seriously impact our ability to live a joyful, happy, and relaxed life.

When I was twenty-one I had graduated from university and like the dutiful student I was I made sure to read the newspapers every morning before going to work to ensure I was up to date with all the latest news. One morning I remember feeling worried and anxious at whatever I was reading. I glanced up from my breakfast, noticed it wasn't yet 8 am, and thought to myself, *it's too early to feel like this*. With a minor sensation of guilt looming over me, I made the decision to stop reading the newspapers every day, and my mornings got a whole lot easier. This was before smartphones, which now enable us to constantly access news and information despite the time of day. Back then I didn't have a steady stream of media and news being directed straight at me through a device that was almost always on my person. Rather, there was some degree of choice about ordering the newspaper, it being delivered, and then reading it. There was a nice ritualistic feeling about the whole thing, sure, but it was also pretty easy for me to let it go. If in that situation today I was using my phone to check in on the news, I have a feeling it wouldn't be quite so simple to quit.

Phones are always with us, always on, and always distracting. Unlike the prehistoric days of landlines, which required no attention apart from when politely ringing, mobile phones command our continuous attention. In my reasonably short lifetime the way we communicate, research, become informed, make contacts, and find entertainment has rapidly changed. It's too early to really know the long-term impact our mobile phone use, our social media consumption, or our reliance on technology have, but certainly it feels almost impossible to write about anxiety without writing about technology.

Story telling—and addiction making

Technology allows us to communicate and tell stories, something humans have done since the beginning of time, but the technology we use today is more highly sophisticated than anything we have seen before (yet in the not too distant future will seem so primitive), and with neuroscientists working alongside computer programmers, there is a somewhat murky shadow behind the seductive and shiny face of social media and the web. Beyond stories of fake news and the improper use of data, the addictive quality of technology combined with its genuine usefulness for completing everyday tasks from buying train tickets to checking the weather means it has become a staple part of our daily lives, and there are now new generations of people who can't remember, or imagine, a day without it.

Whether we crave the latest smartphone, insist on keeping on top of our emails, or spend precious time crafting the best shot for Instagram, there seems to be increasing evidence between the link of social media use and anxiety (check out Google Scholar if you want to get all academic about it), although at the time of going to press it hasn't been recognised formally as a medical condition. We can see signs of social media anxiety within ourselves when we rely on social media to boost our self-worth. Getting lots of likes or new followers can feel like we are being validated for who we are, and we can become reliant on this as a way to fuel to self-esteem. Sadly, these highs are always short-lived and before long we're seeking for the next update to post, the next hit of validation. This also comes when we check for new texts, WhatsApp messages, emails—anything to make us feel needed.

Beyond social media, the 24/7 access to information can give the impression that we should, at all times, be "up to date" with world events, as if by hearing every car crash update or latest political scandal or global corruption story we somehow are better off. I do not mean to encourage apathy or disengagement but too much information could be a bad thing especially given that the information we receive usually has an agenda behind it beyond to inform. The more news we watch the more we teach ourselves that the world is a bad, scary place to be and that people are evil, corrupt, or power-hungry. We start to look for the worst in people, and miss out on all the kindness that is being shared every single day.

You may feel you have a healthy relationship to social media and technology, but it is my opinion that a "digital detox" every now and again is incredibly healthy and restorative whether we feel anxious or not. On my retreats I let guests use their phone as they will, although I do encourage people to try to be more mindful by pausing before they pick up the phone, and to consider if they really need to. It is amazing how difficult this can be in the moment, but how beneficial it can be by the end of the retreat. Stepping away from our phones is for many of us an act of stepping back. When I start to feel anxious, I often distract myself by picking up my phone. This never ever helps and so I have learnt that a few days away from technology clears my mind, calms me down, and helps me actually understand the anxiety rather than trying to push it away. Whatever the problem was, my phone, as smart as it is, is unlikely to have the answers.

Anxiety can stem from a desire to want to control, an inability to go with the flow, a lack of faith in life and the outside world. When the outer world seems to be spiralling into chaos then what better way to find control than to immerse yourself into the digital world, where you can carefully arrange the world and your persona under your complete control? Anxiety can be so unbearable that we long to escape it, but if we are able to slow ourselves down enough to understand it, we can begin to see how it is a tool of protection based on the belief that we are unsafe.

This belief gets confounded when we create more stress in our lives by living at a frantic pace, and neglect any form of reflection, contemplation, or stillness. Society is changing, how we live, work, and eat is changing, and without some time to reflect on the changes that we see happening and to observe how the changes around us are impacting our own lives, we miss the opportunity to see ourselves as part of a great tapestry, as part of the continuous evolution of humankind. It is this sense of understanding and knowing that while it doesn't give us the much longed-for control, it does give us a sense of perspective and awareness that brings a much greater sense of rootedness. We come to see everything as changing, and we find ways to respond to the changes in our own lives. Time for contemplation is so needed in this age of information (information yes, wisdom, maybe not always).

Monkey mind

You may have heard the expression of the monkey mind, a term which originates in Buddhism and describes the way the mind jumps from one thought to another much like the way a monkey swings from branch to branch. The monkey mind can seem like it moves in an illogical and disorganised fashion which can also feel strangely repetitive and familiar. Out of all the hundreds of thousands of thoughts we think every day, many of us find ourselves caught in the same cycle of thoughts, often relating to our fears. It can feel as if worrying about all the possible threats and problems is the mind's default state, but this mindset can shift to a more neutral and balanced place with regular practice of Radical Rest.

Radical Rest can help by bringing stillness to the body and then to the mind, meaning that the monkey doesn't have quite so much swinging to do. This isn't about trying to create an exhausting sense of relentless optimism, but rather about accepting that anxiety is a natural human experience, when we have the tools to respond to it. Isolated batches of anxious thoughts can be helpful—they may help us recognise that we need to do something about the fact that we may be low on cash next month or that there is a problem in a relationship that we need to respond to, but when we get caught in the loop of repetitive, fraught, and negative thoughts then anxiety becomes a greater beast.

Radical Rest is not an overnight fix but with regular practice it can become an aid, an ally, a resource in your life and maybe even in the lives of those around you. I still experience anxiety, and sometimes I feel like it still gets the better of me, but more often than not I am able to recognise my personal symptoms of it (racing mind, need to be busy, wanting to control all the details around me) and then respond by taking the right action (as I mentioned above this includes turning the phone off and monitoring my phone and internet use for a few days, meditating, and spending time in nature). I also find that isolating myself too much in these times can be unhelpful and that I need real face-to-face human interaction. Anxiety can create the illusion that we are alone in this, but believe me, you are never alone in your suffering.

Many spiritual traditions including yoga speak of the human inclination towards suffering and offer practices to overcome this suffering. This shows that while they may not have used the same language as ours, fearfulness has always been around: it's just that the triggers may now be different. Start to understand yourself through journaling, reflection, therapy, or support groups, and it will become easier to understand the experiences that you have as being universal experiences that can actually unite us, rather than divide us.

Soul's purpose

As both stress and anxiety levels in the world seem to increase, it becomes more and more crucial to look at ways to develop our connection with our soul's purpose, not just living to fulfil our material desires. Yoga and meditation can help us to step truly into each present moment, building our resilience and strength. It's why after months or years of practising we can suddenly be confronted with an issue that has lain dormant but now seems to arise out of nowhere. It's almost as though the soul senses that we are now more able to keep sifting through the dirt, and so it gives us the next task in our journey towards understanding. Returning to our soul's purpose, we come back to life after being numb and open our hearts once again.

Technology is only going to form a bigger part of our lives in the future; the news perhaps will veer towards the negative and frightening for some time to come. How we understand ourselves will be essential to using technology to help us create solutions to some of the problems we have created, from the global problem of vast amounts of plastic in the oceans, to the more personal dilemma of how to balance our news consumption. Not only can technology help us create a better future for all of humanity but it can play a useful role in our own lives if our sense of self, our sense of confidence and esteem comes not from needing constant stimulation or validation but from our deeper connection inside ourselves. This is the connection that can really stand the test of time because we know deep down that we are much less in control of our lives and the world than we would like to believe.

If negative thoughts really feel like they are taking over, adopting a gratitude practice such as keeping a journal in which you record the good things that happened that day, or everything you have to be grateful for, can be very beneficial. Even if it is a struggle to find one good thing, try. There is always something we can find to be grateful for, be it the food on our plates or the air that we breathe. Gratitude helps us to connect deeply to our heart space, the centre for giving and receiving love. Like many things, it is a practice, and one which can help balance out the feelings of fear with love. It can break the chain of negative thinking and open us up to all the beauty in the world. I mention this a little more in the Toolkit towards the back of the book.

Anxiety can also be linked with suppressed emotion, or feelings of being overwhelmed or powerless at some point in your life and this is why principle six, community, can be so important. Anxiety is such an isolating condition, but building a community or support network based on a shared interest (such as reading, walking, yoga, etc.) can be wonderfully healing.

How Radical Rest helps

Radical Rest is a way to calm down the body and the mind, and we must work with both. We gain some awareness over our bodies, the areas that feel tight, and the areas that move well. This awareness creates a sense of stability that can reduce feelings of anxiety. The world may seem on the verge of crisis, but we are able to consciously choose how to move our bodies, and we start to notice how we have the capacity to work with our breath.

In yoga we connect with the body and its sensations—we learn to focus our gaze when balancing on one leg, to pay attention to any changes in the breath, and to explore how much of a stretch is possible for us on this particular day. Simply put, yoga awakens our life force, our potential to feel all of our human experience, and to step fully into it, and in restorative yoga in particular we practise becoming still. The stillness of the body helps us to observe the mind more clearly. The quality of slowing down is felt in the slowing down of the heart rate and the gradual lengthening and softening of the breath. Even after one practice we can feel steadier, as though we can think and see more clearly, and anyone who has ever felt anxious will know how appealing that sounds.

From this vantage point we are able to see how the cycle of thoughts changes so frequently and this knowledge may help us realise that our thoughts don't always hold the power or threat they seem to. Anxiety in small doses doesn't have to be a problem. Feeling anxious before an important exam, in planning a big event like a wedding, or when trying to complete an important piece of work on time is perfectly normal, but when anxiety gets out of hand it can start to affect all areas of our lives, as well as our ability to experience joy and love. Much like stress, we are not designed to feel anxious all the time, and worrying about everything that *might* happen is exhausting.

Anxiety is not something we should wish to be rid of entirely, but it is perfectly understandable, reasonable, and possible that we may want to diminish the power it wields over our lives. With Radical Rest we learn how to tolerate our feelings without trying to fix them as we realise they are just messages from our body about things we may need to do differently. With time we are able to find simple pleasure in our daily life and this can bring us great, great joy. To laugh at the sight of dogs playing in the park, to breathe in the scent of freshly cut grass or newly cut flowers, to finding simple satisfaction at spending time making a delicious home-cooked meal—these are pleasures anxiety can so ruthlessly take away from us, yet pleasures which can be restored with the help of Radical Rest. Radical Rest is effective as it helps us to relax our whole being, and when we're relaxed, we're not afraid.

We tend to think of courage as the firefighter running into a burning building, the extreme athlete taking on a new challenge; and yes, there is courage here. Yet I see incredible courage in the efforts of everyday people, in the ability to get up and out of bed and try again, day after day. Courage can be found any time we dare to open up our hearts and say, I love you—especially perhaps when we say it to ourselves. Courage, from Latin *cor* meaning heart, comes each time we allow our hearts to soften, when we pull back the shoulders and stand tall. Courage comes when we tentatively begin to trust when we have been let down before, in the ability and determination to see light at the end of the tunnel, to resolutely remember that it is always darkest before the dawn.

Courage to soften, courage to release, courage to relax; we can cultivate this courage in each Radical Rest practice, every moment we surrender our urge to control and acknowledge our need to rest. Every day we choose to turn off the phone and look up at the world around us to see the beauty in the day we practise becoming more present, more at ease, and more peaceful. Anxiety comes, but we can respond, grounded as we are in the sense of who we really truly are, someone more than our thoughts and more than our body.

Radical Rest

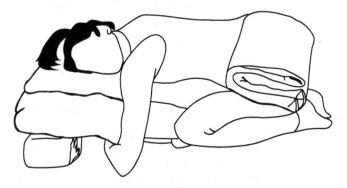

Restorative yoga posture: Child's pose.

What you need:

For this posture make sure you have plenty of padding for beneath your knees. You may like to put a folded blanket on top of your yoga mat. If you have the luxury of two bolsters, you can use two bolsters, creating a T-shape upon which you will lie. If you don't have a bolster, use very firm cushions to create a slight elevation of the bolster the T space positioning of the bolsters as pictured. If you find that the bolsters or cushions are sagging in the middle, avoid the T shape position and instead lie the abdomen flat onto a single bolster. You may also like to place a blanket over your back for extra warmth and feelings of reassurance.

How to do it:

If this is your first time exploring this posture, refer to the preparatory stretches explained on page 40. When you're ready to begin, set up your bolsters and/or cushions as described above. If your bum does not reach your heels then place one or two folded blankets on the backs of the calf muscles, being sure to pull them up tight to your bottom. If the fronts of the ankles feel tight, then roll a blanket and rest the tops of the feet onto the blanket. Take a deep breath in, and as you breathe out, fold yourself over the bolsters, turning your head to either side. You may find an extra blanket for your head is useful if you prefer to look straight down. Stay here for as long as is comfortable, up to ten minutes. Turn your head to face the other direction at the halfway point. This side of your neck may be the tighter side, so if you experience discomfort then turn your head to a more comfortable posture.

Why it works:

This posture is very quieting for both mind and body. The mind draws inward, and the nervous system is soothed. The abdomen softens, the spine gently lengthens and the muscles across the shoulders, back and the intercostal region all relax. This helps us to breathe into the back of the body which is calming for the nervous system and helpful in bringing us back to the present moment.

Watch out for:

If knee pain is a problem, and the suggestions above do not help, try making the height of your bolster higher, so you have less far forward to fold. If it is still uncomfortable, avoid this posture and try one of the other postures suitable for anxiety suggested below. If your ankles are stiff, and the suggestions above do not help, avoid the posture completely, and try one of the other postures suitable for anxiety suggested below. If you are heavily pregnant or in the third trimester, and forward folding is not an option, or simply uncomfortable, then avoid this posture and try the posture given in Chapter 8 on menstrual health (page 138).

Also try:

All of the postures in this book will help to reduce feelings of anxiety. In my experience, it really is a personal preference rather than there being a right or wrong posture to choose. My personal favourites are listed below, but give them all a go and see what works best for you among legs up wall (page 105), relaxation on chair (page 57), and downward twist (page 81).

Anxiety breathing exercise: long exhale, shorter inhale

How to do it:

Before you start, take note of your breath in its current state. Notice if it is faster, slow, steady, erratic. Start by getting settled, lying or sitting, in a quiet, warm place where you are not going to be disturbed for five to ten minutes. You may like to set a timer to help you keep track. Notice how long your breath is, then after 10 to 20 rounds of breathing, start to make your exhale ever so slightly longer, with a soft "haaaa" sound. You may like to breathe in through your nose and out through your mouth. Breathing out through the mouth will help you make the "haaaa" sound. Repeat between 10 and 20 times, or for how long is comfortable. You may like to sit quietly for a few moments after, or if you feel tired, lie down and rest.

Why it works:

Lengthening the exhale is thought to activate the parasympathetic nervous system, and bring about feelings of calmness and stability. This is a simplified version of the pranayama practice vri sama vritti, which refers to a breath where the exhalation is made longer than the inhale.

Watch out for:

With all breathing practices, stop immediately if you feel stressed, anxious, or unwell. Most of us have spent our whole lives not thinking about our breath. To try to force the breath in any way is unproductive. Instead think of this as an invitation to change the flow and direction of the breath. Be curious, and explore what happens. If at any stage you feel agitated, give it up for the day, and try again another day. Anxiety can be complex, and sometimes focusing on our breath makes us more anxious, so be gentle and stick with the restorative yoga posture for now.

Also try:

The breathing practice given in Chapter 6 on stress, as well as the breathing practice given in the section on menstrual health may be effective for anxiety.

Yoga nidra for anxiety:

This yoga nidra for anxiety is a gentle practice, designed to induce feelings of steadiness and relaxation. Access this recording for free via my website www.melskinneryoga.com/free-yoga-nidra and use the password RestIsRadical!

CHAPTER EIGHT

Call to rest: Addiction

A lcohol, heroin, cocaine—we've all seen the stories in the press about the destructive qualities of these drugs, and some of us may have experienced addictions in these areas ourselves or seen loved ones go through battles of their own. We're familiar with this sort of addiction, but we don't hear so much about the addictive daily habits such as coffee, the glass (or bottle) of wine with dinner each night, or the compulsion to stay late in the office every day. We may even joke about these addictions, and consider them harmless. We're still holding down our jobs, relationships and our health is good enough, so what's the problem? We're not really addicts, right?

Well, to answer that let's explore what the word addict means. What images are conjured up as you mull the word over in your mind? Perhaps an image of a heroin addict slumped in a doorway with a needle in the arm or an out-of-control, angry alcoholic stumbling through the streets, perhaps a compulsive gamer, a porn addict, or someone with a ton of credit card debt due to an obsession with shopping. Put simply, someone not like us.

Very often when we think of addiction and addicts, we think of a person with no control and making bad choices, and even if we think ourselves more compassionate than that, and we understand that drug and alcohol addicts have often experienced serious childhood trauma and are searching for meaning or medication through their addiction, we are still thinking primarily in a very dualistic way—that is, we think of us and them. The addict is always "the other." It is not us who are addicted, we believe, it is not us with a problem. Yet there are addiction experts and writers such as Anne Wilson Schaef and Dr Gabor Maté who believe we *all* have a problem with addiction.

The desire to bond

According to the *Collins English Dictionary*, the word addiction refers to the condition of being abnormally dependent on some habit, and the word itself is derived from a Latin term meaning "enslaved by," "devoted habits," or "bound to." Sociologist and director of the Centre for Drug Research in Amsterdam Professor Peter Cohen has replaced the word addiction with the word "bonding" in his work, stating that addictions are simply bonds we humans form and so *what* we bond with is less relevant than the fact *that* we bond.

The human need to bond is biological and our survival really does depend on it. Human babies are dependent on their caregivers for a longer period of time than any other mammal. Without love and care, we would simply die. If the love and care we need, really physiologically, psychologically, and spiritually need, is not there then our brains will look for something else to bond with. To recognise that the drug addict or alcoholic is trying to fulfil an innate desire to bond is to access an empathy and recognition that cannot be found when viewing addicts with disdain or judgement. We are not that different. Perhaps our wine is organic or our food binges done in private, but addiction is addiction no matter what we are addicted to. If we crave it, obsess over it, and feel like we "need" it to get through the day, then it's an addiction.

If we have experienced a form of childhood trauma (a subject I will explore in the chapter eleven) either while still in the womb or as a child, and have not been able to resolve that trauma, then we are more likely to become addicts as we look for a way to replace the connection that was not given by our caregivers, or as a way to numb the pain from the unresolved trauma. Addictions often provide a temporary respite from the pain we may be in, but as we all know, the high doesn't last and too often we are left feeling ashamed, embarrassed, and perhaps already desiring the next hit.

Whilst our addictions are often driven by our innate need to bond, they can too often lead to us feeling isolated and alone. This can make the vicious cycle of addiction more painful due to the way our culture punishes and shames us, and subsequently how we then punish and shame ourselves. By labelling certain addictions as wrong or illegal we have created a moral platform built on swampy ground. To punish drug addicts is to deny them the kindness and love they have most likely been craving whilst our own more legal addictions are encouraged and promoted through aspirational marketing campaigns and economic systems that need us to spend, spend, and spend some more in order to feel successful, happy, or complete.

When we view our addictions as personal failings that could be overcome if we just had enough willpower then we may be misunderstanding our need for those addictions in the first place. If our addictions are driven by our emotional and biological need to bond then approaching bad habits with willpower alone may ultimately become a recipe for failure, and only serve to strengthen any negative beliefs we have about ourselves. Anyone who has tried to give up their addictions or change their habits will know that cravings can be unbearable—just ask an ex-smoker or a chronic dieter!

Cravings, when we give in to them, can feel amazing in the moment, but are swiftly followed by shame, regret, and remorse. We vow never to repeat that mistake again, until of course, we repeat it again, and then we blame and shame ourselves for our weaknesses. Ultimately we are blaming ourselves for our humanness, and while most of us would resist labelling ourselves as addicts, how many of us could give up our addictions easily? Giving up easily means going without the object and not being caught up in the constant thinking, craving, and desiring for that object, so while we may not view our addiction as harmful or particularly negative, the key thing to observe is just how attached we are to them.

The busyness buzz

Addictions serve to keep us busy, distracted, and occupied but one of the biggest (and most socially acceptable) addictions is busyness itself. Busyness is the badge of honour representing our success and wealth. It's as though the busier we are the better we are, as though the more appointments we squeeze in during the day, the more productive and popular we become, even though ironically we risk becoming more inefficient as we try to do too much in too little time, and our friends and family get tired of our flakiness when we succumb to tiredness and cancel engagements at the last minute.

Despite our sense of busyness, research by the Centre for Time Use at Oxford University[1] shows that we are not actually any busier now than we were at the beginning of the millennium, we just feel like we are. Why is this? In the chapter on anxiety we explored the role of technology in creating a sense of urgency and need, but our use of technology is really a reflection of the mind. I think the felt sense of busyness is real, in that we genuinely feel busier than ever, but I also think that part of that busyness comes from a need to belong.

In the same way that our reasons for meeting friends in the pub, coffee shop, or bar are more to do with connection than drinking, being busy helps us to belong in a culture which values output and productivity. Buying certain brands, going on certain diets, and playing certain sports all help us feel as though we belong. We create all of our attachments, be they labelled as good or bad by society, not because we are weak or failing but because we are human and we want to belong.

Work is still my most addictive drug of choice, and it has taken me a long time to see that my desire to work hard and "secure" myself in a high-paying job in an organisation that worked "for a good cause" was really my desire to be needed, a way to validate my existence, and to locate a sense of safety I had lost in my younger years. Because working hard is celebrated in this culture and rewarded with money, status, and power, it didn't cross my mind that this could be an addiction until I started to turn the looking glass on myself and begin to see more clearly. I know myself well enough now to know that this desire comes from a time when I felt very alone, with very little money, and I believed the only way to protect myself was to work really hard. When I now find myself caught in a pattern of working too hard, I review my diary and create some space to "do nothing."

If I am too stressed or agitated to go straight to "doing nothing," I practise the restorative postures of Radical Rest, which help reduce feelings of stress and anxiety and make it easier to slow down. Perhaps most important of all, when I give in to my addictions and overwork or start filling my diary, I treat myself with compassion and understanding, rather than berating or criticising myself. This has to become a regular practice if it is to work over time, and without the compassion I know I will quickly feel defeated and hopeless and give in to the addiction.

Filling the void

Addiction is a way of looking for love in peculiar places. Our parents and caregivers may not have been able to give us the love and care we wanted, or perhaps they were neglectful or abusive. We still crave the feeling of love and connection, so we look for it in other ways, such as through chocolate, sex, and power, and while there is a distinction between a potentially fatal heroin addiction and an addiction to shopping, ultimately what is driving our addiction is a craving that has developed from a need in us that has not been met, the need to be loved.

If so much addiction is caused by childhood trauma, which can start as early as in the womb, then it becomes more important to move away from blame and towards understanding. When we understand that our parents, like all humans, are doing the best that they can in the ways they know how, we can start to see how their trauma may have been passed to us, but also passed to them by previous generations. We can start to see how huge the scale of trauma is, and just why we are all addicts because really our addictions are our natural response to an essential desire in all our hearts, the desire to be loved and to love. Love is so crucial to every layer of our being. Whilst it is a big step forward to think of addiction as a disease rather than as a personal failure, there is still a need to see addiction as an intelligent response by the body and mind to find a way to survive, a way to find some substitute for love in whatever way it can. Seeing addiction in this way takes us away from the "them and us" mentality, and instead invites a kinder and more nurturing approach to viewing addiction.

Many addictions may stem from childhood trauma, but I believe several also come from our sense of disconnect from our bodies which we have been told are unholy and full of sin, our disconnect from each other as we increasingly become sold on the idea of individuality, and ultimately our disconnect from who we truly are, that is whole, beautiful, and creative beings with endless capacity to heal, love, and be loved in return. When we start to realise our own power in facilitating our own healing we start to realise how important it is to feel our own pain in order to transform.

While we ourselves play the most important role in healing (healers therapists and practices like Radical Rest are just the tools we choose to use), we most certainly cannot and should not do this alone—connection and community are essential here. We can build a community of friends, colleagues, therapists, and more, we can connect with our surroundings, and with nature, and ultimately connect to a form of self which is beyond the material world, beyond our ideas of who and what we are.

If we believe that drug and alcohol addiction is something that can just be given up, we may be right, if we find something else that fills the hole that the drugs and alcohol were filling. For me, the more I began to surrender my sense of egoic self to my yoga practice by giving up the career that had defined me, giving up the drive to have a different body to the one I had, and giving up the beliefs that made my body hard and rigid, the more I found that my bouts of binge eating abated. In times of stress and anxiety, I may find myself searching the fridge for something that wasn't in there, but I have developed the self-awareness to observe this better, and try to respond.

Renounce and enjoy

It was Gandhi who was reported to have said "renounce and enjoy" when asked the secret of his life in three words. Some speculate that he was referring to some lines from the ancient Indian text the Upanishads, where there is a line "Rejoice in him through renunciation."[2] In these words Gandhi encapsulates the joy that can come from indulging in the pleasures of life without needing them. Practising Radical Rest will help you to reduce the cravings in your life while bringing you more pleasure from a glass of wine with friends or a few squares of really good chocolate. You may find that other habits, such as too much TV, porn, or shopping simply don't bring pleasure any more and so they fade away of their own accord. You may even discover a new contentment in deep rest, and a freedom in realising how little we really need.

This isn't about giving up the small pleasures in life, but rather about cultivating your awareness of your relationship with those pleasures. Do you really enjoy drinking coffee every morning or is it just a habit that brings you a feeling of comfort or energy? Why are you picking up your phone right now? Do you really want a Netflix marathon just because it's Friday night? The more we become honest with ourselves about our habits, the more we can assess whether they are truly bringing us joy, or whether we have become addicted to them. This is a form of awareness, of paying attention and noticing yourself.

How Radical Rest helps

Addiction can also be created as a way to find fulfilment outside ourselves, or to numb the pain we feel inside ourselves. Any compulsive behaviour, any "devoted habits," take us away from the actual feeling in the body, which means we move out of the present moment. The brief dopamine hit we get from our addictive habits cannot substitute for a deeper, longer-lasting yet more subtle feeling of wholeness. The quality of wholeness can be found through the journey of connection. The word yoga itself means to "yoke" (it's often translated in a more accessible manner by the word "union") and although yoga practice is ultimately a way to connect, to yoke, with the Divine, we can also see it as a way that we start to connect with our bodies, our breath, our minds, and each other. All yoga including Radical Rest helps us to develop compassion for others as we start to see past the superficial barriers of gender, race, age, and nationality, and see something deeper within us, the soul in each of us.

This can sound like a big ask, and in all honesty, it is. Seeing the humanity in everyone is very, very tough, especially in those who have done you wrong. Ultimately, though, it is the pathway of compassion and forgiveness that can help us grow, and it's always a good idea to start with yourself. When I started to see that some of my behaviours were addictive and that the need to be addicted was coming from a part of me trying to connect, I quickly realised that berating and criticising myself for my own addictive tendencies was futile and misguided and instead I started to become curious and compassionate about my actions and cravings. I'm not saying this was easy and the desire to criticise myself often overtook the need to understand myself. However, understanding that bonding is a vital part of our human existence, can help cultivate our understanding of the true scale of problem, and why some of the principles of Radical Rest, such as compassion, curiosity, connection, and consciousness can help.

We are cultivating greater presence through the practice of Radical Rest. If we are using our addictions to fill an emptiness inside us then we can use yoga nidra as a way to start to explore the bodily sensation of emptiness, as well as use our imagination to bring in the opposite sensation of fullness. We are not becoming attached to one or the other, rather we are exploring the possibility of experiencing both. We start to develop a more curious nature towards our feelings, rather than wasting our energy trying to push them away or resist them (which is far more exhausting than just being with them). Because we relax our way into yoga nidra, it becomes far easier to explore our sensations, particularly the more uncomfortable ones, than if we try to do the same when we are tense and stressed.

Rather than using Radical Rest as a way to quit or overcome our addictions, we instead use it as a way to help us slow down and become steadier. In this state of relaxation we can better see our desires and cravings, and over time develop the ability to choose what we do in that moment. When we choose to rest we are also choosing self-acceptance. We no longer need to keep ourselves distracted but we find more ease in being present. Even difficult emotions become easier to sit with, and so rather than focusing on "beating" our addictions (which keep our mind in the future) we choose to accept ourselves as we are in the present.

When we welcome our whole selves and allow ourselves to just be, we discover the true meaning of power. It doesn't always feel safe, conditioned as we are to feel fearful and ashamed, and it doesn't feel familiar, but it can become safe and familiar with practice. When we refuse to accept ourselves we get caught in a battle of believing we're not good enough, and start a never-ending battle to change and control ourselves. The battle is exhausting and fruitless because if you believe you are broken then there is no drug, no product, and no self-help book than can fix you. The only "cure" for feeling broken is to connect with the stillness within you that recognises that you have never, for one moment, been broken in this life.

The regular practice of Radical Rest cultivates awareness, and also deepens your capacity to be comfortable with not only slowing down and relaxing, but also exploring your capacity to feel the spectrum of emotions we humans experience. Over time, it becomes easier to accept periods of discomfort and suffering, and from here we can enjoy our habits, rather than being held hostage to them. In fact we might find our pleasure in those habits becomes greater the less we crave them.

Be compassionate, be curious, maintain a sense of humour, and enjoy. Our time on this Earth is short, and precious. Let yourself be human—but let yourself be Divine at the same time. You are not here to work your life away, you deserve more pleasure than an extra slice of cake can bring, and all your cravings are trying to bring you back to love. Let yourself indulge in Radical Rest for no other reason than that you can.

Radical Rest

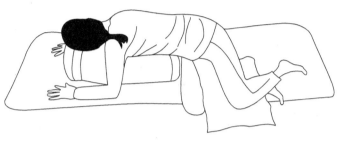

Restorative yoga posture: Downward twist (in Sanskrit, adho mukha jathara parivartanasana).

What you need:

This posture can be done with just one bolster or firm cushion, but can also be done with up to three. You may like a blanket to cover yourself with, plus a blanket or thin cushion to support the head.

How to do it:

Sit on your right hip, facing the long edge of the mat. The bolster should be placed next to the hip, with the narrow edge of the bolster closest to your hip. If you are using two or three bolsters, make sure that your hip is roughly lined up to the middle of the bolsters. You may like a blanket folded in the place where you head will land. Start with an inhale, and sit up taller. As you exhale begin to turn your belly, ribs, and chest towards the bolster. Then lower your abdomen down onto the bolster, as though your belly button were trying to lie flat on the bolster (it may not actually do this, but this is the direction you are moving in). You can turn your head to face in either direction, but turning away from your knees will be a stronger twist for your neck, so if your neck is stiff or you are nervous about overly twisting the neck, then keep your gaze the same direction as the knees. In the beginning you may like to practise for just one to two minutes on each side; with practice you can build up to ten minutes on each. Move slowly between transitions, and rest on your back at the end of the practice.

Why it works:

By twisting the spine we embody the idea that we need to change shape, to see things from a different perspective whilst uniting all the different parts of ourselves. We are able to relax the body down onto the bolsters, allowing ourselves to be held, while we patiently wait for change to happen. This is an important message when we are dealing with addiction: to be patient, and kind, and persistent with our progress. Restorative yoga can teach us new ways to soothe our bodies and minds, and many drug and alcohol recovery centres now use yoga and meditation as ways to support people in substance addiction recovery. Physically this posture stretches the muscles between the ribs (the intercostal muscles), relaxes the back muscles, and improves the flow of blood to the back of the body. This helps to create space in the back of the body for the breath, which is deeply relaxing.

Watch out for:

Be mindful of twists if there are lower back or sacroiliac problems; move cautiously, and if necessary seek the advice of an experienced yoga teacher. If you have a shoulder injury, make sure you have plenty of support under that arm, particularly around the collarbone area. If you are pregnant, avoid any posture which involves twisting the spine and the back of the pelvis. Later on in pregnancy it may also be uncomfortable to fold forward. Instead try the posture given in the chapter on menstrual health (page 138).

Also try:

This posture works well as part of a yoga sequence. You may like to start with all the preparatory postures on page 40. Twists work well in-between a forward folding posture and a backward bending posture. After the preparatory postures you might like to take child's pose (page 68), then the twist on both sides, followed by a more backward bending posture such as the bridge-on-chair on page 93. This should leave you feeling calm yet energised. For a quieter practice, do the bridge-on-chair first, then the twist on both sides, and end in the child's posture. If you don't have the time or inclination for a full practice (the sequence mentioned above could be done in about thirty minutes) then choosing either a forward bend such as child's posture will calm you, and a backward bend like bridge-on-chair will energise you. Both of these postures can be practised in isolation.

Addiction breathing exercise: lion's roar

How to do it:

Start by observing your breath in its current state. Notice if it is faster, slow, steady, erratic. Then sit comfortably. You need to sit, rather than lie. Kneeling can be good, with the knees wide and the hands on the thighs or the floor, but if kneeling is uncomfortable then sitting cross-legged or on a chair is fine. Try to keep the spine long (rather than hunching over the chest) if you can. Once you are in a comfortable seated position take a couple of deep breaths. Drop your chin to your chest, then when you inhale (breathing in through the nose if possible), lift your chin to the ceiling. You may like to close your eyes. As you breath out, stick your tongue out, and make a roaring sound (like a "haaaaaaa" sounds). If you closed your eyes, then open them wide as your exhale, looking out of the far corners of the eyes. As you come to the end of the exhale, replace your tongue in your mouth and look straight ahead. Repeat up to five times. You should feel energised after this practice but try not to rush around or sit up too quickly.

Why it works:

This is a lot of fun! It can help us relax, giggle, and let go of any tension we may be carrying, especially in the throat. We feel more courageous (like the lion) as we make strange noises. It can give us a sense of fresh-ness, and an ability to start each day afresh. It can help us find our inde-pendence (you might not want anyone watching!) and bring some heat and energy into the body.

Watch out for:

With all breathing practices, stop immediately if you feel stressed, anxious, or unwell. Most of us have spent our whole lives not thinking about our breath. To try to force the breath in any way is unproductive.

Instead think of this as an invitation to change the flow and direction of the breath. Be curious, and explore what happens.

Also try:

Often our addictions stem from a desire to control. You may like to try the balancing breath, given on page 59, in the chapter on stress, as a way to balance out cravings and desires. If you are feeling particularly tense, try the breathing practice given in the section on grief or the section on anxiety. Both are effective in creating space in the body, and calming the mind.

Yoga nidra for addiction:

A slow and steady recording, this yoga nidra helps you to explore holding different sensations and feelings. Access this recording for free via my website www.melskinneryoga.com/free-yoga-nidra and use the password RestIsRadical!

CHAPTER NINE

Call to rest: Depression

Everyone from the Dalai Lama to Fearne Cotton to the World Economic Forum seems to have an interest in our happiness, and perhaps rightly so when according to William Davies, author of *The Happiness Industry*, one third of adults in the US and almost half of adults in the UK believe that they occasionally suffer from depression.[1] It seems as if everyone's got an interest in *fixing* depression, but with a subject this vast and complex, is fixing depression even the right language? Should we first be getting to the heart of why we feel depressed?

I remember hearing a story about a woman who was going through a difficult divorce and had two young sons. She went to the doctor to help with her low mood. She was put on antidepressants. There was no conversation about the events in her life which may have resulted in feelings of depression, no conversation about how diet, exercise, and moral support could help, and in the average twelve minutes that British doctors reportedly spend with each patient, it is unlikely that much of a meaningful dialogue could have really taken place. This is just one story of someone's experience with depression—there are of course countless stories, from different people of different ages, races, genders, sexuality, nationality, and religion. One thing many of these stories seem to have in common is the prescription of antidepressants.

The drug effect

Since the 1980s at least, depression has been treated with pills, and in order to be prescribed antidepressant medication, we must believe that depression is a medical condition to be treated. Walk into a doctor's surgery today and you could be diagnosed with many forms of depression including seasonal affective disorder (SAD), major depression, bipolar disorder, premenstrual dysphoric disorder (PMDD), post-natal depression, manic depression, and several more, and the likelihood is that you will receive some form of antidepressant medication.

It is beyond the scope of this book to explore the effectiveness of antidepressant medication, but it does seem odd that there is so much money being made from antidepressants and yet so many people still feel depressed. Could there be more to depression than a case of out-of-balance brain chemistry? Books such as *Lost Connections* by Johann Hari, *Why Zebras Don't Get Ulcers* by Robert M. Sapolsky, and *A Mind of Your Own: The Truth about Depression and How Women Can Heal Their Bodies to Reclaim Their Lives* by Kelly Brogan all offer science-based insight into why the drugs might not work (or at least may not provide the whole solution).

In yoga, depression, like anxiety, is something experienced in both mind and body. The heaviness in the body, the dullness of the mind, the lack of desire to do anything, and the inability to experience any sense of joy are some of the qualities associated with depression. Some people may find these sensations are alleviated through medication and so therefore consider the medication to be a help, but many people also remain on this medication for life, alternating between levels of dosage while never quite feeling safe or ready to give up completely. It is appealing to think of something as simple as taking a pill every day as helping us to combat what can feel like a suffocating weight, yet without the understanding that comes from our inquiry into our depression, can we ever be free from depression? Perhaps the question is *should* we ever wish to be totally free from depression? The answer to this is not a simple one, but let's look at the concept of happiness as an end goal, and why this may be an impossible hope.

The happiness dilemma

Understanding happiness is not just for the Lamas and Fearnes of this world. Research into happiness takes place within the studies of neuroscience and sociology, sometimes on behalf of advertising and market research. We live in a time where it is believed that we can understand what makes us happy by collecting data, and boy are there huge amounts of data to mine, accessible for those with money and vested interest. We voluntarily give away information about ourselves all the time, including on social media where we share not only our photos and memories but also our emotional status. To those who believe that happiness can be measured by a smiley emoji, we are living in a dream age of information.

In 2014, the then UK Prime Minister David Cameron chose to measure the UK's happiness, cue much derision from commentators. Yet Bhutan, a country which has been measuring happiness since the 1970s (rejecting GDP, gross domestic product in favour of GNH, gross national happiness), has attracted much positive attention from the rest of the world for its philosophical approach to policy. Regardless of the motives behind political desires to measure our happiness, I wonder, what if happiness is something which cannot be measured at all. What if happiness—as well as depression—is far more individual and personal than we can rationally understand? What if all our emotions and feelings are subjective, rather than objective, abstract rather than material, and we as human beings are more complex than the posts we share on social media would suggest? What if happiness is not even the right word? What if our natural state of being is not dancing on the rooftops all year round, and what if my idea of being happy is completely different to yours? How can this be measured? Regardless of the philosophical and scientific debate that surely lingers in the arena of measuring happiness, happiness is being measured.

Freedom

To have the desire to measure something implies the desire to not only understand but also control that thing. If we can scientifically state what collectively makes us happy, then there is no reason for any individual to be miserable, right? And if there is no reason to be miserable then it is easier for us to blame individuals for their malaise, rather than to examine the external influences around that person, such as their upbringing, health, and socio-economic status.

If there is a formula to happiness, then why let power struggles, racial tensions, and wealth inequality get in your way? Within spiritual circles, the belief that you attract everything which happens to you grows ever more popular with a population who long to believe they are in total control of their lives. Of course our attitude and beliefs have a huge effect on how we respond to situations and the choices we make; but to fall for the fallacy that each person is fully and wholly responsible for every single event of their life is akin to saying that the victims of the Holocaust had it coming, that cancer patients are somehow to blame, that it's all karma anyway so why worry? Easy to say when you're white, rich, and drinking a soya milk latte after your yoga class, hey?

In parts of the yoga tradition, happiness is not much discussed as a potential goal or outcome. There is a notion of contentment, which upon contemplation is not really like happiness at all. My understanding of this complex and ancient tradition is that happiness is not the goal, but freedom is, the freedom to make choices in your own life and the freedom to understand the essence of your being, regardless of race, gender, or sexual orientation. What if there was a way that helped us find contentment in our lives without deluding ourselves in the meantime? To even contemplate these questions requires an individual to feel some sense of personal power and self-esteem, because if you don't have either of these then to consider the idea of freedom can seem pointless, frustrating even. I know, because I was that individual.

As someone who has experienced what I consider mild depression on and off throughout my life, it took coming to yoga to begin to see that my depression was linked to my childhood experiences of grief and loss. I started to recognise a connection between why I would fall into such dark spells when on the outside my life looked well. I started to develop a compassion for myself when I realised that just because people around me would tell me how well I had done, I would still feel full of self-doubt, separation, and at times, self-loathing. Importantly, I began to see how much our culture places value on the notion of perpetual happiness and how this could actually exacerbate the experience of depression. As if being depressed isn't enough to deal with, we pile on guilt and shame for being depressed in the first place, as though we personally have done something to cause this situation.

The more yoga books I read, from philosophical translations of books like the *Yoga Sutras* to more contemporary research into health, wellbeing, and spirituality, the more I began to develop a new relationship with depression, and that word "relationship" is key, because without first trying to understand our depression we are trying to fix or ignore something that needs our attention. We live in an age when happiness is the goal and depression is a problem to be fixed with a pill, but what if depression is a symptom of an imbalance, and not the cause? What if depression is more than a disease, but a messenger, something which wants us to wake up and pay attention? And what if the drugs don't work, at least, not when prescribed without any conversation around one's social support network, financial situation, sense of power in the world, or belief in something greater than this physical world?

The story beyond the sensations

Our high stress, fast-paced lifestyles are creating chronic stress and the busy-ness culture leaves us relying on far more caffeine and sugar than is necessary, sending our hormonal system into a spin and leading to a roller coaster of emotion. We've already looked at the mind-body connection, and when it comes to depression, what we eat definitely affects how we think and feel. A diet high in sugar and low in essential vitamins and minerals is thought to disrupt blood sugar levels, affect digestive functioning, upset the thyroid gland, and cause inflammation. Not only this but an overload of gluten and dairy products may cause the healthiest of meals to have little impact if the gut is unable to absorb nutrients from food.

Equally a lack of exercise, fresh air, and natural light can all have a negative effect on us, as well as stressful life events, such as loss of any kind. We are affected by the external, of course we are, but we also have more control over the internal, our inner landscape, than we realise, and this realisation could be an essential key to supporting ourselves with our depression. Depression can keep us locked into a gloomy and dark inner world which may seem full of dead-end tunnels clogged with mud. If we can learn how to light a match in the darkness we can start to see the shadows for what they are, shapes which are cast when the light is obscured.

When we cast a light onto our emotions and sensations we step outside the experience for a moment. The more we do this, the more we start to recognise our patterns. We might remember that our depression started when we were about fourteen, at the same time our father lost his job and we were made homeless. We might begin to realise that we often hear ourselves being highly critical towards ourselves and others, and this leads us to feeling isolated, lonely, and depressed. The more we develop this awareness, the more able we become at changing the thought patterns that create the criticism, the more we may realise that the childhood trauma which seems to have taken place in a different lifetime needs to be processed and resolved, so that we can let go of the baggage we've been carrying around for so long, and step into the new world.

When I used to try to pretend that the sad times had either never happened, or that they had had no impact on me, I was actually more frequently depressed than when I started the work of carefully delving into and exploring these locked-away emotions. I created space, I developed my awareness, and I was able to become more objective in my understanding while very much letting myself grieve for all that seemed so long ago.

Community, compassion, consciousness

Many people feel a lack of community around them. We often leave our childhood homes for work, move house frequently as students and young people, change jobs more regularly and never get to know our neighbours. We may find we feel we have more in common with people we meet through the web than the people we grew up with, and this may be true. The nature of community is rapidly changing, and as we become more reliant on ourselves, we struggle to find reasons to get to know one another. Yet community and human contact is so essential to our well-being.

We also need compassion. Human beings are more fragile than we admit, and more resilient than we know. We can confuse resilience with stoicism, pride ourselves on being able to endure pain and suffering without a word of complaint, and then when the dam of crammed up emotions finally breaks, we can cry bitterly at our weakness and failings. Compassion helps us to accept our vulnerability and our need to ask for help. Ultimately we need to elevate our consciousness, because it is by elevating the mind that we realise our connection to something within ourselves that is beyond our feelings of depression.

Consciousness gives us a new way of thinking, of feeling, and importantly, of responding. I know from my own experiences of depression how difficult it can be to respond in the midst of a dark spell. The heaviness, the lethargy, the sense that everything is pointless: all feelings that make it difficult to do anything at all. We can and do get stuck in depression which is both unbearable to experience and awful to imagine.

We must practise making conscious choices every day to develop our sense of personal power. This isn't necessarily about making a right or wrong choice, but simply recognising that when we choose to have tea or coffee, we are making a choice. Choosing to spend our lunch hour at our desk or outside in fresh air is—for some of us at least—a choice.

Sometimes if we are depressed it can be hard to find the enthusiasm to do anything at all, so even picking up this book is an achievement and very much worth acknowledging. Although the thought of getting out of bed can feel as impossible as flying to the moon sometimes, every action that we take to help ourselves has a positive impact. The key is to start small, taking one step at a time, and each step is to be taken with love and acceptance. If you can't get out of bed and into the shower, can you get out of bed to open the curtains? If you can't make it onto your mat to practise, can you at least make it onto your mat, if just to sit or lie?

There is always an action you can take, no matter how small, and you may feel like it's not making any difference, but I promise you it all adds up. One day at a time, and it will be worth it because yoga almost always makes us feel a bit better straight away. It offers us hope. It provides light at the end of the tunnel by bringing the balance our bodies constantly seek to our biochemistry and our endocrine system. It releases muscle tension, encourages full deep breathing from the diaphragm, and begins to undo old patterns of holding and tightness. Simply put, it helps us relax and makes it safe to feel again.

Sometimes we avoid our feelings because we think they are bigger than us, when the truth is we are so much bigger than our feelings. We worry we will be overwhelmed or swallowed up by our feelings of darkness, loneliness, and depression, but the reality is that we are stronger and more powerful than we give ourselves credit for. The dark patch you are going through will not only pass but could also offer inspiration and hope for others. It may bring you greater compassion so you can learn to listen and allow others to share their story. It could release you from your cage so you can truly build a connection with yourself and with others—and in doing so, find yourself on a path of awakening, of acceptance of yourself and new ideas about who you really are, a beautiful purposeful soul with a real reason for being here.

Imagine a world where we were told hopeful and positive stories of human kindness (of which there are in abundance), a world where collaboration and discourse between politicians was encouraged, and we celebrated a sensitivity and understanding around human vulnerability.

The systems that run our world have denied our essence and so our soul lives have become dismantled and our connection to God made accessible only through organised religion, rather than through our own bodies and minds; and so we have become disconnected from ourselves as a source of wisdom.

Yoga helps us connect with ourselves by removing toxicities in body and mind. From a yogic perspective depression is an imbalance of the energetic flow of life force around the body. By experiencing depression that life flow, which brings us hope, energy, and joy, is disconnected, and we feel like we have been cut off from the source. By practising yoga, we are able to reconnect to a source of energy which can help us over time to discover that although we may *feel* depressed, we are *not* depression itself. Depression is our experience, but it does not define us. With each yoga practice that we take, we learn a little bit more about how to be with our experience, but not be overwhelmed by it.

How Radical Rest helps

Yoga helps to teach us that everything is in a constant state of flux, and Radical Rest helps us develop our understanding so we can absorb these teachings and integrate them into our own life more fully. While the practices in this book have been designed for you to practise easily at home and alone, I cannot emphasise enough the importance of building a community with others. Perhaps you have a friend who would like to join you on an exploration of Radical Rest, or your family members would like to share the practices? Perhaps there is a yoga class near you that may not be Radical Rest but could offer you the chance to practise and get to know other people? Radical Rest is as much about the nine principles as it is about the practices I share at the end of each Call to Rest chapter. In this case, community, compassion, and connection could be some of the key ingredients to begin to move forward and out of the dark night.

Radical Rest is an incredible act of self-care. Because of its gentle and relaxing nature, we avoid the risk of punishing ourselves with yoga. A common error is to go to a yoga class which is too advanced or complex for our needs, and to push ourselves too hard, resulting in injury or feelings of inadequacy, meaning we miss the point of yoga entirely (which is to connect more deeply with ourselves, not to sustain unhelpful thought patterns about ourselves). Whilst I am not proposing that

Radical Rest is a cure for depression, I do suggest that certain qualities of the practice could create a container for the depression to be held in.

Incidentally, while Radical Rest yoga can work wonders for some with depression, it may not always be the best for everyone. I find that although restorative yoga is effective for my "dark days," yoga nidra is not, at least not when doing it alone. Working with a yoga nidra teacher, however, is different, as we draw on the sixth principle of connection. For me, to lie down with my eyes closed and enter into deep stillness on my own is not as helpful as taking an energetic form of yoga in a group, preferably with a friend or two. Because of the diversity and complexity of depression, I encourage you to explore what works for you. If your depression is heavy, sluggish, and lethargic, then more vigorous uplifting activity may be suitable on some days more than others. Specific restorative yoga can help, including postures which lift and elevate the chest, giving us more space to breathe fully and deeply. I have chosen such a posture that I feel helps us to both calm down and re-energise, bringing a greater sense of balance to the whole being.

Radical Rest helps to bring more light into our hearts and minds, and if we can find even the slightest smidgen of hope that we are worth taking care of then we can find light at the end of the tunnel. The more we can understand, believe, and feel hopeful, the easier it becomes to take each day as it comes. We come to understand that we are part of a much greater tapestry than any of us could ever imagine, and this realisation can be likened to lighting a candle in the cave of depression.

Radical Rest

Restorative yoga posture: Supported bridge-on-chair (in Sanskrit, setubhanda sarvangasana).

What you need:

This is another posture requiring the use of a yoga chair, but if you do not have one, you may be able to substitute an ordinary chair or even the side of the sofa. It is important that the backs of the legs are fully supported, and that you can relax in the posture. You may also need a blanket to lie on, a blanket as a pillow, and a blanket on the chair seat if using a metal chair.

How to do it:

Take a bolster or firm cushion and place it just in front of the chair seat, making sure there is about a hand's width distance between the bolster and chair seat. Sit on the bolster, sideways on, then carefully swing your legs one at a time on the chair seat—be sure to use your hands to support your weight. Lower yourself backwards carefully until your upper back is on the mat, and the back of your pelvis is on the bolster, with both legs on the chair seat. You can also practise this with the bolster vertically on the mat, so that the narrow edge of the bolster is at the base of the shoulder blades.

Why it works:

This posture elevates the legs above the heart, which is thought to improve circulation. It also relieves lower back pain, brings a gentle stretch to the back of the legs, reduces feelings of fatigue, and opens the heart space. Yoga teacher Tias Little likens depression to cigarette smoke, describing it as "shroud[ing] the lungs."[2] If we are able to open the chest, we expand the capacity of the lungs to open, and encourage the flow of prana, or life force, through the body, increasing our sense of vitality and energy.

Watch out for:

If you find the posture is pinching the lower back, try smoothing the flesh of the buttocks down by pressing your feet down on the edge of the chair seat, lifting your hips slightly, and using your hands to push the flesh down. Please note you must be fairly strong in the core in order to lift the legs and lower yourself back. If you are nervous at all, please do not risk doing this at home alone, but find an experienced teacher to guide you. In the meantime, you can practise without the bolster, so the legs are still lifted but the whole of the back is on the floor. Or you can try one of the alternative postures suggested below. If your lower back is still pinching, there may be tightness in the upper back, in which case try turning the bolster into a more vertical position as described above. If you are still experiencing tension in the back, then discontinue and explore one of the alternatives suggested below. This posture may not be suitable during menstruation.

Also try:

Other uplifting postures which open the lungs include the receiving posture on page 138, and legs up the wall (with bolster) on page 105. If you are heavily pregnant or menstruating avoid this posture and try the posture given in the chapter on menstrual health (page 138).

Depression breathing exercise: long inhale, rapid exhale

How to do it:

Start by observing your breath in its current state. Notice if it is faster, slow, steady, erratic. You may like to bring some steadiness to the breath before beginning by taking the breath awareness exercise given on page 123 in the chapter on trauma. When you feel ready, sit comfortably. You will start by taking a deep breath in, then a short sharp breath out. Repeat this up to 25 times. The emphasis is on the inhale being longer than the exhale. This is a version of the traditional yoga breathing practice known as Kapalabhati (meaning skull-shining). Once you have finished 25 breaths, either stop there if that feels enough, or repeat for another 25 times, taking up to three rounds. You should feel more energised and awake at the end, but do not rush to your feet. Make sure you feel steady and balanced before coming to standing.

Why it works:

It is thought that a longer inhale may help with depression by activating the sympathetic nervous system, the one responsible for the fight or flight mode discussed in the chapter on stress. This may seem unusual at first, but if practised in short bursts could bring a new sense of energy into the body. It can be extra effective if taken after a cold shower.

Watch out for:

With all breathing practices, stop immediately if you feel stressed, anxious, or unwell. Most of us have spent our whole lives not thinking about our breath. To try to force the breath in any way is unproductive. Instead think of this as an invitation to change the flow and direction of the breath. Be curious, and explore what happens. Do not practise this if pregnant or menstruating.

Also try:

Depression, like anxiety, is complex, and so as always explore with the practices on offer, and see what suits you best. The practice given in the chapter on stress may bring a sense of balance to the system. If any of the breath practices start to make you feel sluggish or heavy, stop.

Yoga nidra for depression:

This short and sweet yoga nidra offers a journey directly into the light and love of the heart. Access this recording for free via my website www.melskinneryoga.com/free-yoga-nidra and use the password RestIsRadical!

CHAPTER TEN

Call to rest: Grief

Death is the moment that the life force leaves the body, which it inevitably will do at some point. Grief however is often for the ones who are left behind and whatever it is that grief has to teach us, it is not a lesson many of us willingly choose. We do not know the destination, or the distance we must travel, and it is a long and unpredictable journey which can be a very lonely experience. No matter how supportive our friends, families, and colleagues are, no matter how shared our grief is, there is still a part of grief which is very much our own. We may be one of many siblings who lose a parent, but that loss is still unique to each of us. It is personal to the core, and our ability to properly mourn affects our ability to acknowledge the loss. It felt right to me to include grief in this book, because although it does not fall into the same category of illness, disease, or imbalance in the way stress, anxiety, depression, and addiction all do, it is a form of suffering which, strangely enough, can be alleviated when we actually let ourselves suffer with it.

A journey begins

I remember sitting on a beach in Western Australia, aged twenty-four, knowing a flight home awaited me, feeling so physically aware of the distance between myself and England, and knowing I couldn't go back. Not yet. I ended up away from home for over a year and had one of the best years of my life, but it was also that year that I started the process of healing. It took being on the other side of the world to start this journey. Seeing the world, opening my eyes and mind, and giving myself space just to be allowed me to relax, but ultimately it was the journey inwards that opened me to the inner landscape of my being, to discover the trauma, grief, and pain that lay within. Travel helped me find my place in the world, but it was finding yoga and spiritual practices and gradually committing more and more to these practices that ultimately were my recovery.

Looking back on when I first came to yoga I had no idea of really why I was there. This was before yoga was as popular as it is today, and in fact my first experience of yoga wasn't even really a yoga class, it was termed Body Balance and was a combination of yoga, tai chi, and Pilates. When the class was finished, I got into my car to drive home and burst into tears. After a few minutes, I stopped crying and drove home, wondering what that was all about. I was twenty-one, impatient and inquisitive about the world around me, and not at all aware that I had huge amounts of grief and pain in my body, and so my self-inquiry went no further, but it is clear to me now that that was just the beginning of a long and what sometimes seemed a very slow path towards yoga. I didn't know it at the time, but each time I practised yoga I was redeveloping awareness in my body and creating new neural pathways. I was, unknown to myself at the time, learning how to feel safe again. I had been operating from my head for so long that learning to open my body was sometimes a difficult process. My shoulders were tight, and my hips were numb. In fact I didn't even realise how tight my hips were until it came to practising pigeon pose during a yoga teacher training weekend, a strong hip opener that you usually remain in for at least a minute. As I struggled in extreme discomfort with the posture, I glanced at my fellow trainees for sympathy, only to see everyone seemingly sinking their pelvis to the floor with ease. My perception of my body at this point was still as something to change, alter, fix, something that was at odds with the marketing material I saw around me, and thus something undesirable in its present state. It took a lot more yoga and a lot more discomfort before I began to connect the tightness in my body with the rigidity in my ability to fully express myself.

My path to becoming a yoga teacher is still a wonder to me. Although I signed up for teacher training I had no intention of being a full-time teacher, or even a teacher at all. My career was my anchor, job titles, big organisations, and salaries being my salvation. I had no sense that teaching yoga was something I wanted to do, let alone any belief that it could actually provide an income, but gradually I taught more, and worked (in a conventional sense) less, until teaching yoga, alongside sharing other practices like reflexology and astrology, became my main work and my purpose in the world, and this could not have been possible until I let myself fully and completely grieve, and by that point, I had a lot of grieving to make up for.

The grief that eventually led to yoga started when I was very young. My mum had died when I was aged two and as my father wasn't around my Nan and Grandad had been my guardians. My Nan was the centre of my world, and the anchor of my family. When she died I was aged fifteen, and my world alongside my Grandad's fell apart. At the funeral, the church was packed out, and I think there were even people outside the church, unable to fit inside but still wanting to pay their respects. The whole funeral my jaw was set solid. I knew that if I was to cry, I would not just cry but I would collapse and weep and wail, become inconsolable and, the terror of all Westerners, out of control. I also knew this was not what we did in church, that here we mourned in a more private and dignified way, and whilst I am not condemning that in any way, for me, it was not what I needed as a teenage girl, a frightened child. And so I swallowed that pain, that fear, that heartbreak deep down inside me, and carried it around for a good fifteen years.

I do not blame anyone for this, I do not blame our culture or our society, I do not blame the church, and I do not blame anyone else, but I do believe that the rituals we have created to help a body leave this world may not always help the ones who get left behind. I wasn't able to experience my grief until a long time after both my grandparents had died. Instead I diverted my attention to figuring out how to pay bills and buy food on a limited income and making my way to university, where I discovered a love for learning. I loved how studying made my world become bigger and stopped me thinking about myself, and so university led to travel, which eventually led me to Bristol, and after a few more personal ups and downs, I found my way to yoga, and that is when I finally started to grieve as I learnt to explore moving and opening my body in new, often awkward, ways.

Although I had spent years avoiding my grief, through yoga it began to emerge. I found my emotional responses to yoga postures becoming strong, and my bouts of fatigue seemed to increase, even though I was doing less. This is often referred to as the "healing crisis"—although we put ourselves on regimes and plans which we know will make us feel better, we often don't realise that before we feel better, we have to feel worse. This is because our traumas are held on a cellular level—that is, they are not just experienced in the mind but experienced in the body. When we start to release the traumas, we are "resetting" the nervous system back to a healthier state, but we have to go through the release first. Because my experiences of grief and loss had been so extensive, and I had held on to them for such a long time, I believe my healing crisis was particularly strong.

In order to feel my grief, I needed some space. Until that point I had filled my adult life with intense amounts of activity. I literally never rested. From early morning starts at the gym, to having more than one job at one time, to filling my weekends with training courses, I lost the habit of simply sitting with a book, taking a nap, or gazing out of the window. Whilst I don't regret a lot of the activities that I did, I recognise now that I was keeping myself busy and distracted so that I didn't fall into the dark hole of grief. And that is what grief can feel like.

Unexpressed grief can easily become depression and over a prolonged period of time can change our biochemistry by reducing serotonin and norepinephrine and increasing production of cortisol (one of the stress hormones). It can even cause our hippocampus to shrink, the part of our brain which stores our memory,[1] not to mention the shadow it can cast over the rest of our lives if left unresolved. Part of my journey towards supporting my feelings of depression was to let myself feel the grief that I had carried for decades. While this wasn't an easy and straight-forward journey, I believe that by allowing my feelings to emerge to the surface, they were then able to dissipate and I was able to move forward in my life, creating space for more love and acceptance. Even now I have moments of sorrow and sadness over what I lost, but I am far more comfortable and able to deal with these emotions now than at any other point in my life.

As I increased the frequency of my yoga practice, and immersed myself in the study of yoga philosophy, I became more aware of the connection between my thoughts, my emotions, and my body. I started to wonder why child's pose used to leave me in tears, and realised over time that I was so highly stressed and exhausted that child's pose was the only time I actually let myself stop trying so hard. It took me a long time to reach this realisation, but as I gained more experience in my practice and by sharing yoga through teaching, I started to learn more about the emotional effects of postures, as well as the physical. I saw through my own experience as well as the experience of clients and students just how remarkable yoga was at supporting emotional health as well as the more well-known physical benefits it brings.

Modern day grieving

In the UK there is no statutory law that permits someone to take paid leave in the event of a bereavement, although in 2020 there should be a new law called the Parental Bereavement (Leave and Pay) Act which entitles a parent who loses a child under the age of eighteen to paid leave. Beyond this, your employer is not legally obliged to give you time off when you are grieving. In the US, grieving can now be considered a medical illness (and therefore treatable with drugs) if you are still "unhappy for more than two weeks after the death of another human being."[2]

Any of us who have felt grief—be it from the loss of a pet, person, much-loved job, or home—know that the experience of grief is much more complex than this. While we may have absorbed the notion that beyond a funeral and wake and with a handful of days off work (if you're lucky) we should then suddenly bounce back to "normal," our bodies and hearts know that there is a new normal to get used to, a normal that takes more than a few days off work, a normal that involves that person or situation not being there anymore. Life does go on, but our experiences of the world cannot help but be changed, just as we ourselves are changed.

When we let ourselves grieve we are also giving ourselves permission to cry, to be sad, and to feel lost, and this makes it a remarkable gift. Whereas most of the time we are told to think on the bright side, grief allows us to explore the dark. When we understand that this is OK, that being sad is as valid as being joyful, we can experience grief as a pathway to deeper empathy, compassion, and a desire to live a more meaningful life, be it through our actions or simply in our thoughts.

Grief doesn't really leave us, but our experience of grief changes as time moves on, and a night of endless sobbing can suddenly shift to a bright blue sky the next morning with an inexplicable sense of hope. You can go years feeling perfectly fine, then a song or an image or even a yoga posture can conjure up a memory which takes you right back to the heart of grief, right back to that moment of realising there has been a loss. It's like time travel: one minute we are enjoying a nice stretch in yoga, and the next we are hiding our tears.

When we are moving through intense grief, we can get exhausted. If we live in the shadow of grief such as the grief unexpressed within our families for example, then we can become heavy in body and mind. Rest can help by rejuvenating our whole being, and by allowing us to slowly reconnect with the totality of feelings. We may also grieve for what *didn't* happen in our lives. For the children we did not have, the relationship that did not come, the hopes and ambitions left unrealised. We carry not only our personal grief for our own losses and what-could-have-beens, but also a collective grief for what we see being lost, be it the takeover of corporate entities on our high street, the loss of precious plant and animal life around the world, or the sense of grief we feel for humanity in the wake of terrorism or war. This sort of grief serves to remind us just how fleeting and precious our time on this Earth is, and causes us to contemplate our lifestyle and behaviour in a way which may bring around positive change.

From one form to another

Science is starting to prove what mystics have known for centuries—our body is not an innate object that we drag around with us, rather our bodies are a source of multidimensional and intelligent information which are highly sensitive and always changing, moment to moment, day by day. The nervous system affects the physical body, and the endocrine system affects all aspects of our growth. The breath is vital not only in its ability to keep us alive, but in our ability to digest and eliminate food and improve the steadiness of our mental and emotional states. The more we realise just how alive we truly are the more we can celebrate the preciousness of our time here and honour the process of grief. Death of another reminds us of our own mortality, reminds us that we too will die and the world will continue. This is terrifying for the ego. Even spiritual people get sick, yoga teachers can get cancer, and bad things happen to good people.

There is suffering in the world, and our spiritual practices have the potential to teach us how to move through our own suffering and to love and support the struggle we see in each other, but oh my is it tempting to use the spiritual path as a way to avoid, avoid, avoid by believing that we are somehow "above all of that." The spiritual path is a path of transcendence and transformation. To transcend literally means to go above a limit or expectation and is derived from the Latin *transcendere*, meaning to climb. To transform means to move across, through, or beyond one form to another. While we work to elevate our consciousness to that of a more spiritual path, we cannot use this as an excuse to ignore or "go above" the suffering we see in everyday life. Rather we learn to see the suffering, and to acknowledge it. We may not be able to solve homelessness, we may not be able to bring about world peace, but we can learn to acknowledge each other's pain and grief. This requires us to be vulnerable, as we open our hearts to another's suffering and admit we cannot fix their pain.

Vulnerability is tough. It's not an easy place to be, and for many, it is not a safe place to be. I still have moments of panicking over leaving my career for what can feel like a financially insecure vocation. Interestingly, if I am able to stay present with the panicky feelings, they lose their power somewhat. I notice that, like all emotions, they rise and fall. As I maintain my breath, I gain a clarity of mind, and can see through the fog of panic that not all my worries are worthy of a reaction.

What do we do in those moments when we are overwhelmed and feel a sense of loss? We allow time and space. We remember our compassion and we direct it protectively towards ourselves. When we are able to feel the devastation of grief, we are also able to feel the full power of love because we are grieving for what we have loved. It is through these experiences that we see the gift that grief has to offer, as well as the pain, a gift to the vulnerable state of being which may not be culturally validated or appreciated but which allows us to really become present, to become ourselves, and to be here, in this life. Not constantly busy with goals or plans or dreams, but to just be right here, right now.

If you'd asked me to believe this ten or fifteen years ago, I would have thought you were insane. The idea of hope and faith would have felt foolish and naive as I struggled to support myself, believing that there was no one there to help me. Grief as a form of love would have felt as insulting as the idea that emotions want to move through us felt ridiculous. I urge you to feel any frustration, despair, and disagreement with this chapter! Share with me your thoughts, your reflections, and your ideas. Grief is a strange creature; I am sure she visits us all in different ways. Whatever you do don't reject your grief, don't push it away. When the time is right, the grief will begin to emerge, the icy protective layer will begin to melt, and the pain will ask to be felt.

How Radical Rest helps

I personally have often thought how the love of my grandparents carried me through the difficult times of later years. Even though they died when I was at a very vulnerable age, I was able to feel the love they had shown me later on in my life. Long before I had any interest in spirituality I thought that the love and stability of my childhood had created something so steady that it got me through loss and grief. Developing my yoga practice and working with spiritual healers and shamans helped me not only to think that thought but to really, truly feel it. And it started with Radical Rest, and the feeling of being safe enough to relax.

Radical Rest creates space for any suppressed emotions or feelings to come to the surface by releasing tension held in the muscles and helping us to breathe again. It becomes safe to feel into our bodies, and let our emotions fully express themselves. Radical Rest lets us heal the exhaustion, to tentatively and gently begin to access the present, enter into the sensory experience of being human. By using yoga postures to see our mental patterns and to embody qualities that we may avoid or suppress, which for some will be strength, resilience, determination, or willingness to change, and for others could be softening, releasing, relaxing, and trusting, we can truly believe that we are whole. When we use yoga simply to build up our one-sided ego, and take our compulsive and driven force onto the yoga mat, we are really missing out on something beautiful. We miss out on the beautiful gift that yoga offers—that is, to feel whole.

Radical Rest

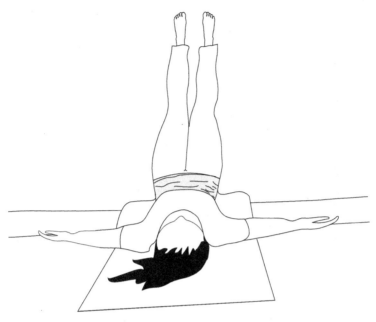

Restorative Yoga posture: Legs up wall (in Sanskrit viparita karani).

What you need:

You will require access to a clear wall. Use of a bolster or firm cushion to place under the pelvis is preferable, as it is the elevation of the pelvis and the expansion of the chest which is effective in relation to depression and fatigue, such good companions of grief, but it is possible to enjoy this posture without these. It is recommended to place a thinly folded blanket under the back of the head.

How to do it:

Place the bolster approximately one hand's width away from the wall. Sit sideways on the bolster and then use your arms to support yourself as you lift your knees from the floor towards the chest, and swivel yourself towards the wall—this is the tricky bit, and you can lose your balance. If you are new to this, or nervous, then start without the bolster. Once your legs are up against the wall straighten them as much as is comfortable. Adjust the blanket beneath the head so the folded edge of the blanket is touching the neck but not on shoulders. You can stay here anywhere from five minutes to twenty. If you are new to this posture, start off for smaller periods of time, maybe for five minutes. Come out of the posture by bending the knees towards the chest, rolling to the side, and slowly pushing yourself up to sitting. If you are using the bolster, roll completely off it and lie on your side on the floor. Don't be in a hurry to get to your feet.

Why it works:

In traditional Chinese medicine the lungs are associated with grief and the heart is associated with love. This elevates and opens the heart and lungs, our centres for joy and sorrow, love and grief. This allows us to safely feel our emotions, whilst in a calm and relaxed state. If you find that tears begin to flow, you can stay in the position, but you may find tears gathering in the ears. If this bothers you, slowly come out of the pose, but allow your tears to continue and subside naturally. The elevation of the legs offers deep rest and recovery from fatigue, which can accompany the process of grief, and may also emerge when we have unexpressed grief within the system. This is a great way to lift your energy and spirits, especially if you can't force yourself to attend a yoga class. It's also an effective posture after travelling or sitting for long periods of time as the elevation of the legs and feet supports the circulatory and lymphatic systems. It's very refreshing to feel the tension draining away from the legs and head, and, spreading the arms, open the chest, thus creating the perfect counterpose to being hunched over a computer screen. I used to enjoy doing this when I came home from a day in the office. I lived in a tiny flat at the time, so I would lie on my bed and put my feet on the wall at the place where the headboard should have been.

Watch out for:

If you find it hard to completely straighten your legs, you can keep them slightly bent. When the hamstrings are tight then it can be a little tricky getting into this position using the bolster. Instead, try this posture without the bolster so that the back of the pelvis is on the floor rather than elevated. Once you become more familiar with the posture and feel more comfortable in it, you can then try it with the bolster. The positioning of the bolster at the wall is a delicate one. I usually suggest having it approximately a hand's width away from the wall or skirting board. If it is too close to the wall, then it becomes more challenging, especially if the hamstrings are tight. Equally too far away from the wall will put a strain on the pelvis—if you are unable to place your legs up the wall and keep your bottom relatively close, then try shifting further away from the wall, bending the knees, and placing the soles of the feet against the wall. This may also be a good alternative if you have lower back pain. Tying a yoga strap around the thighs may help if you feel like your legs are splaying apart. Not recommended for menstruating women, women more than three months pregnant, or women at risk of miscarrying. If this applies to you, then turn to page 138 and try the posture for menstrual health.

Also try:

I recommend the posture in the menstrual health chapter on page 138, which is also a wonderful way to support the grieving process as it allows the heart to fully open and creates a wonderful feeling of being held. If you are struggling with fatigue as a result of grief, then please feel free to explore all the postures shared in the book, and see what works best for you.

Grief breathing exercise: belly-heart breath

How to do it:

Start by observing your breath in its current state. Notice if it is faster, slow, steady, erratic. When you feel ready, bring your awareness down to your belly. You may like to place one hand on your belly. Notice that as you inhale your belly rises up into your hand. As your exhale, the belly retracts, flattening slightly. Once you feel comfortable with this, you may like to make the breath a little longer. With a longer breath, again inhale down into your belly, then feel breath move up into the heart space. It's as though on an inhale the breath starts deep down in the belly, then expands up into the centre of the chest into the side ribs. On the exhale, the breath moves back, in towards the heart then back down into the belly. It is a bit like a wave, like the tide gently ebbing and flowing through your body. Count ten of these breaths, then pause, allow the breath to return to normal, and continue if you are enjoying the practice. You may like to sit quietly for a few moments after the practice is over, or if you feel tired, lie down and rest.

Why it works:

This breathing encourages us to breathe fully and deeply. Breathing down into the belly exercises the diaphragm muscle, which is an essential muscle in the breathing process. This breath will bring fresh oxygen into the blood and encourage a more efficient circulation process. We are "holding on" to our breath and also holding on to our emotions: this breath will invite some movement. As a result, we may feel emotions rise to the surface. This is perfectly OK, as long as you feel safe. If you feel overwhelmed at any point, please stop, and rest.

Watch out for:

With all breathing practices, stop immediately if you feel stressed, anxious, or unwell. Most of us have spent our whole lives not thinking about our breath. To try to force the breath in any way is unproductive. Instead think of this as an invitation to change the flow and direction of the breath. Be curious, and explore what happens. In particular, if you notice that your breath is the other way around (i.e., as you inhale your belly retreats, and as you breathe out, your belly goes up) then don't go any further. Try the restorative yoga posture given for the chapter on trauma. Practise this for some time, then try again with the breath. This is known as reverse breathing and is very common, but we would want to restore the breath to its natural rhythm before controlling or manipulating the breath in any way.

Also try:

Simple breath awareness, as explored in the section on trauma, page 123. Sometimes if we are frozen in our grief, this can be enough to produce a flood of tears or other emotion. If this happens to you, know that this is not a bad thing, but if you feel too overwhelmed, come out of the practice, and if it feels suitable, write down your experiences or share them with a sympathetic friend.

Yoga nidra for grief:

A quiet journey back to feeling, through stillness. Access this recording for free via my website www.melskinneryoga.com/free-yoga-nidra and use the password RestIsRadical!

CHAPTER ELEVEN

Call to rest: Trauma

Trauma not only has many forms and has many labels, but affects many of us, in many different ways. From the war veteran returning home to the person abused or neglected as a child, the after-effects of a distressing event can outlast the experience itself and disconnect us from the reality of our present moment and the possibility of our future.

Yoga is a practice which can help us connect to the present moment by increasing our awareness of our body and our breath, both of which are only in existence in the here and now. Through yoga we become more conscious of how a posture can change the way we breathe, of how a thought can trigger a physical response, and how regular practice can change the choices we make each day. Through yoga it becomes easier to tolerate uncomfortable sensations. It becomes easier to be present.

Author and trauma expert Bessel van der Kolk's research has shown that yoga is one tool which may help trauma survivors reconnect to their body after trauma has disconnected them.[1] This can be especially powerful for anyone who has ever felt unsafe in their body, such as the victim of sexual abuse or assault. Learning how to move and feel your body can be very empowering for anyone who, for whatever reason, stopped feeling their body a long time ago. Yoga also can help us to reduce the effects of stress, particularly by moving us out of the fight or flight response.

As well as fight or flight, the body and mind have a third resource to help us manage an overwhelming experience, and this is known as freeze. When we have experienced a stressful situation, and been unable to fight or flight our way out of it, we freeze. This is described by Dr Peter Levine as a feeling of helplessness, a feeling of having one foot on the brake and the other foot on the accelerator at the same time.[2] We are primed to take action yet we cannot, and so we "freeze" as a way of numbing our bodies to whatever may be taking place. While this may be effective in the short term—we feel less pain, for example—if we are unable to "defrost" after the event is over, or if our stress is coming from the ongoing stress of, say, paying bills or the fear of losing our homes, then we may remain caught in the fight-flight-freeze response.

When we numb our body, we may be preventing ourselves from feeling pain, but we may also be cutting ourselves off from feeling love, compassion, empathy, and joy, to name just a few emotions. When we don't want to acknowledge our pain, we cannot begin the process of understanding and acknowledging our experiences through both the mind and the body, and without any acknowledgement we cannot move forward in our lives. Living in a constant state of fear prevents us from giving and receiving love, and we can begin to feel isolated and alone, sadly at a time when we may most need support.

It can be easy to become numb even if we don't feel we have been subjected to a specific or isolated traumatic event. Our sedentary lifestyles, sitting for hours at a desk or in a car actually causes our bodies to ache, but if we have to do these things for our survival then we might choose to ignore the messages our body sends us. We may also want to numb our emotions because we feel embarrassed or ashamed of them. We don't want to appear out of control or weak, we don't want to bother other people with our worries, or we might feel critical of ourselves for feeling less than well.

Becoming numb can feel like a protection, or a way of managing ourselves. We may feel that we can hide the "unacceptable" parts of ourselves, but actually by protecting ourselves we harden, carrying a heavy coat of armour throughout life, creating tension in our physical body as we literally try to keep things out, and bringing disconnection to our emotional body as we refuse to express the flow of emotions that move through us. This is not often a conscious choice but a condition called alexithymia, where we do not have the words to express our emotions.

For many, many years I was unable to express the well of deep grief and sadness that was within me for all that I had lost. I spent many years pretending my grief did not exist and that the tumultuous events of my younger years had had absolutely no effect on me—and *I believed this to be true.* When I look back to the younger me, I can now understand what was happening. I understand that, on one level, she genuinely believed she was fine, but I also understand that she had no other way to survive that situation. It was when, many years later, an important relationship ended and I was again thrown in disarray with nowhere to live that the previous trauma finally began to release.

It took being completely overwhelmed for a second time to begin to feel all the emotions from the past. I had also started practising yoga. It may be hard to believe, but I genuinely see that breakdown of sorts as an essential part of my spiritual growth and mental and emotional recovery. It was only through losing everything all over again that I was ever going to find myself on this path of healing, growth, and transformation. It is essential that anyone healing from trauma of any kind works with their body as well as their mind. Working with the mind alone takes us so far, but to really begin to heal, we must begin to find safe and nourishing ways to work with the body.

Yoga and trauma

In recent years there has been an explosion of yoga therapy offerings, and I myself have described some of my classes and workshops as therapeutic and healing. I use these words to refer to the health-boosting states of relaxation that yoga offers. Relaxing the body boosts the immune system, balances the endocrine system, and helps us to breathe more fully, taking us out of fight or flight. In this sense, yoga can very much feel like it's helping us to heal as it returns our body to homeostasis, essentially meaning balance. Every day we may get knocked out of balance—a stressful day at work, a poor night's sleep, an argument or conflict with a loved one—and this is why we return to yoga regularly, to restore and rebalance ourselves.

Yoga helped me cope with my grief and stress after experiencing emotional upheaval and distress throughout my childhood. My teachings went on to become more emotionally focused, taking me into areas such as depression and anxiety and yes, trauma, although this was never particularly planned or expected. I had one especially powerful experience working with a woman, who kindly shares her story here. I asked her to share her story for this book, but she actually went on to share it with a far greater audience, as she goes on to explain herself.

After attending one of my Restorative Afternoon workshops, three hours of restorative yoga and yoga nidra focused on freeing the breath, Kim approached me to enquire about the possibility of one-to-one work for PTSD. We went on to work together for over a year, and the change that I have witnessed in her has been incredible. I sought her permission to share this story, but actually she'd already done that herself. Kim suffers with complex PTSD (c-PTSD) as a result of a severely abusive childhood. Sexually abused for years by her stepfather, emotionally abandoned by her mother, and assaulted by other men, Kim has suffered in ways most of us cannot begin to imagine.

She is incredibly bright—a human rights lawyer in fact—as well as being gentle, kind, and empathetic. Our sessions together have gone deep, have sometimes been dark, but have also been full of fun and laughter. I have watched Kim work so much on healing her symptoms of c-PTSD and in finding out what brings her the sense of wholeness. She has built herself a community, taken control of relationships, and brought poetry, nature, and self-care practices into her life. In essence she has created Radical Rest in her own life, before I even developed the principles!

She may have received support from me, her doctors, and her friends, but ultimately she has done this work on her own, guided by her incredible sensitivity and innate wisdom; she knows what she needs to be well and whole, but she can only access this when she knows she is worthy. And how many of us, even with seemingly idyllic childhoods, truly know this? And how many of us do the work to find this? Kim made some big decisions during the time we were working together. She set up a Meet Up group for women in the Bristol area who had been sexually abused. She contacted the regional daily newspaper, the *Bristol Post*, to see if they would perhaps advertise the group, and somehow found her way to a very kind journalist who was moved by her story. Together, Kim and this journalist created an article which would involve Kim removing her anonymity.

According to the journalist, to waive the right to conceal your identity is very rare in the case of child sexual abuse stories (understandably so), and Kim was told that the story may attract interest from the national press if she went ahead with this. This could have affected her whole life, including her career, but she decided to go ahead. She wanted people who have been abused to find their voice, and so the story was published and subsequently picked up by the *Mail Online*. Kim was also contacted by the NSPCC to support their campaigns, and published another article in *Cosmopolitan* magazine. Kim bravely refused to change her Facebook profile, keeping it public so people could find her, and she was flooded with messages from women sharing their stories, their pain, but also their gratitude and love. Even the comments below the article online (which we all know can be a place for hatred and abuse) were an outpouring of love. I still work with Kim occasionally, and I have a huge amount of respect for her. I am humbled by her magnificence and honoured to be able to work with her in such a close way. Here is her story.

I first met Mel at a restorative workshop she was holding called "Find your breath." I was finding life increasingly unbearable and I had resolved to throw myself at every kind of "healing," however weird and wacky, as a last resort. My emotions were so unmanageable and pain so overwhelming, that I had given up on life. I thought I would have one last-ditch attempt at finding an "answer" so that when I finally took my own life on my 30th birthday, it would be safe in the knowledge that I had tried everything and no, it wasn't going to get any better. This was my "grand plan" to alleviate my guilt that I wasn't trying hard enough, that I was being pathetic. I wonder if Mel had known this on the day I walked into her class, what she would have said.

I knew I was terrible at breathing into my tummy, often holding my breath or shallow breathing, consistently on edge, so when I saw the workshop on breathing advertised, I signed up. I am not a yogi, or at least what I thought a yogi was. I am not defined, or bendy, and my hair does not slick back into a ponytail. I rarely go into Sweaty Betty for fear they will laugh me out of the shop and I hate kale. So walking into my first workshop, I was apprehensive to say the least. I gritted my teeth and expected to be judged and was excited to get the whole thing over with.

I will try not to turn this into an "Ode to Mel," but it is an understatement to say that Mel carries with her a wisdom and authenticity I have rarely experienced before. Suddenly, I was in a room where it was OK to just ... be. Something in the way Mel held the space gave me permission to exist, and to put down my load. Being around Mel gives me the same feeling I get when I walk into a beautiful forest or see a beautiful landscape and I exhale, not realising I have been holding my breath. Permission to stop pretending, I suppose. I sidled up to her after the workshop, which I had wept and slept my way through, and asked about her one-to-one work.

When Mel first came to my house for a one-to-one visit, I could not close my eyes in front of her. Lying down in front of her was excruciating even with my eyes open. I was so exposed and what if she was looking at me, judging me, laughing at me. As you can imagine, Mel was beyond patient, creating extremely short nidras that lasted only a few minutes with my eyes open, focusing on the surroundings of my own home. And from there, my exploration of yoga nidra grew.

Very shortly after starting one-to-one with Mel, my precarious world finally crashed and I had a huge breakdown. I was put under the care of a mental health crisis team for a month. I remember one appointment with the crisis psychologist extremely vividly. I was expecting him to tell me the magic cure, the miracle answer for the horrendous symptoms which had recently been explained to me as complex PTSD. "There is no answer," he said. "There is no cure or 'treatment'. You just have to work out what makes you feel safe. Find what makes you feel safe, and keep doing that."

It isn't an exaggeration to say that at that point, in my memory there was only one time I had ever felt truly safe in my body in my life, and it was during a yoga nidra. I remember Mel saying to me during the nidra, "Is there anything you need to do at this moment, anywhere you need to be, any questions you need answered?", and knowing in my whole body that there wasn't. That at that moment, everything was OK. Mel often repeats to me during a nidra the words "You cannot get this wrong," words that are slowly becoming a mantra for my life. Through nidra, I have been able to find a place where I can recognise that although my feelings and emotions may be in the middle of a huge storm, that it may hurt like hell and everything may feel so wrong, that underneath all of that pain and anguish and loss, all is well. I hesitate to use the word soul as I don't want to alienate those who don't believe in the concept—but I have learnt that whatever I am going through, my soul is well, I am well, and that it will pass.

Having had mental health problems for most of my life, I have always thought of myself as desperately deficient. I have sought answers and cures to try and "fix" myself. To be better, to be more normal, less ... me. Make myself whole. Yoga nidra is the first practice I have come across that starts off by saying—"No, no, you are whole already. You are perfect just as you are. You might not feel very perfect and there may be so many symptoms you want to change, but you aren't broken, you are whole and all is OK." This, combined with constant reassurance that there is no wrong way to do yoga nidra, has allowed me to access a place where I really do feel whole.

The other aspect of yoga nidra that I am so grateful for is that I finally have a self-care tool that works for me. Many many mental health guides these days advocate self-care and rightly so. They often come with a recommended list—bubble baths, chocolate, a manicure, shopping, a magazine. Treat yourself! Absolutely none of this would work for me. Shopping was a nightmare, a balance between my brain saying if you buy this you will look better and more people will like you and you will feel better, and worrying about money, and convincing myself I was too awful to wear whatever it is I was buying. Hot baths had a similar effect—I would lie there tense, thinking how awful I looked naked and wondering how long I had to stay in the bath for and why my muscles were still so tight. Finally, I have something that makes me truly feel rested, really, really rested, because I have a way to feel peaceful. It is the first time I have found a way to let my body let go and relax.

It has also been a way that I can access what I am feeling much more safely. The rising panic of "Oh my god, I'm about to feel something and it is going to be awful and I will go crazy. How can I stop this?", that so often led to self-harm, now has a new narrative. "My feelings cannot hurt me. Can I give it a name? Where in my body can I feel it? It can't hurt you, just relax into it," has led me to such a greater understanding of my emotions, where they are coming from and where it hurts. When you know what you are feeling, and that it can't hurt you, it is so much easier to figure out why you are feeling it, have a good cry for it, or rage, and let it go.

I don't believe in miracle cures—and neither does Mel. Yoga nidra forms part of my armoury now, along with psychotherapy, antidepressants, spending as much time as I can outdoors and being with friends. It won't "fix" my c-PTSD. But it has allowed me to rest where I am, whole, which has given me the energy to keep going, given me the strength to get to psychotherapy in the first place, given me the comfort blanket to put on after psychotherapy when it leaves me in bits. It tells me I am worth it, that I deserve to be here and that I can always come back to this place of safety. Without that as a foundation, I truly believe that none of the other things would be possible.

Kim's story is incredible, and her courage in sharing it is something I think many of us could benefit from because even if we don't think of ourselves as having experienced trauma in any particular way, many of us are still carrying the weight of the British stiff upper lip (which may include those of you not British but with antecedents from the UK). Sharing our experiences helps lighten the burden we may have been carrying all these years, and in doing so inspire others to do the same, as we come to realise that we are never as alone as we believe we are.

Remember Kim's story, and know that you too have that courage within you. When we keep rediscovering our feeling of wholeness, we can really love ourselves in that moment, and from here we can truly heal and transform. Terrible things may have happened to us, we may need a whole toolbox of supportive tools from medication to meditation. Radical Rest can help as it invites us into a deeper realisation of who we really are. While yoga nidra might not be suitable for everyone (going into a trance state may not be helpful for someone who is already really good at dissociating—if you are experiencing a diagnosed form of trauma or working with a therapist of any kind please seek guidance before starting yoga nidra), it can, as Kim and I myself both experienced, be incredibly supportive for others. For me, it was probably one of the first times I truly rested, and I cannot describe to you how truly wonderful that really was.

Radical Rest also promotes finding community, connecting not only with like-minded folk but ultimately seeing your connection with the people around you, your work colleagues, your neighbours, the man or woman working in your local shop. It is a journey towards seeing a connection with everyone and everything around you, not a journey of insta-healing that requires you spend thousands of pounds and attend luxurious five star retreats. It can sometimes be hard to see the link between practising yoga on your own and connecting with the person walking down the street in front of you, and perhaps there is some science that explains why, but I know from my own experience and the experience of clients, fellow practitioners, and books that many, many people find that yoga opens their heart in a way that cannot help but lead us to see the world around us in a more interconnected way.

When yoga may not help

There are times when certain types of yoga don't help people with trauma. If the teacher of that particular style of yoga insists on postures being a particular way rather than allowing the practitioner to explore their way into a posture, this can take the practitioner away from their felt experience, and put them in a passive role, which is probably unhelpful and could create a feeling of shame, particularly if their trauma related to an experience where they felt passive and were being dominated, or if they already feel uncomfortable in their bodies. It may also increase feelings of failure and ineptitude if they are called out for "doing it wrong," and reiterate the message that the body is a problem which needs to be corrected, especially if the teacher offers physical adjustments without prior permission.

Being in a busy class can feel stressful if there is not enough space, and being surrounded by very fit and able yoga practitioners can also feel intimidating, especially if people are wearing very little, as may be the case in a heated room, for example. That's not to say that any yoga that does offer physical adjustment, that is hot, or fast, or directive is bad or wrong in any way, but that in the context of trauma, it may not always be suitable. We human beings are incredibly complex organisms, and how one person feels about a particular yoga practice can be entirely different from another, and yet neither is wholly right or wrong. Reconnecting with the body helps us to check in with our gut instinct a little more, and helps us make decisions about what is right or wrong for us.

Radical Rest also aims to promote feelings of worthiness, rather than the inadequacy or embarrassment we may fear when going into a yoga class. Radical Rest is not the sort of yoga that gets you hot and sweaty, meaning that you don't need to wear skimpy or revealing clothing, and Radical Rest aims to support and hold the body, rather than you trying to contort yourself into uncomfortable and awkward shapes, which for someone with trauma may exaggerate or encourage feelings of failure.

Radical Rest helps us to feel the healing power of yoga, not just discuss it or think about it. We can readdress the emotional balances in our system, as well as the physical ones, so as well as healing chronic pain and tension we can also begin to heal insecurity, low self-esteem, and constant worrying. By removing the stress, we can feel again, and as such, "defrost." Radical Rest is also a form of self-inquiry. Dropping into a deeply relaxed state can help us access feelings in the body more easily, even if they may be described as unpleasant or uncomfortable. We develop what is known as witness-consciousness as we learn to accept all our sensations and feelings, without labelling anything as good or bad or right or wrong while remaining present. Our ability to recall painful emotions from the past while staying rooted in our present being can be very effective, although is not recommended without the support or guidance of a professional therapist.

When I teach yoga nidra in a class setting, I generally avoid doing too much in the emotion/thought realm and keep the class more rooted in experiencing their body and breath. This alone can be tremendously valuable and avoid mistakenly upsetting anyone. We of course also take ourselves out of fight or flight every time we practise, thus helping us to calm down and feel safe again, and we may even be creating new neural pathways. Research on neuroplasticity explains just how the brain is capable of changing itself based on your external environment, so if you can make some changes to your environment, like resting more, you may actually be able to change the structure of the brain.[3]

How Radical Rest helps

Radical Rest opens us up to the possibility of presence, of getting comfortable with having "nothing to do," and finding safety where there may not have been safety before. Ultimately it is the relaxation of Radical Rest that helps us to feel safe, and it is feeling safe that takes us out of fight-flight-freeze. By learning how to feel the body, we start to recognise the signs of fight-flight-freeze more and more in daily life. The more we can become "rooted" in our bodies, the better able we are at responding to immediate and real threats, including things that can occur every day, such as cycling around a busy city and navigating buses and cars, or being startled by loud sirens (two things I regularly experience!). We may not always be able to stop the external situations which can upset us, and possibly trigger a "flashback" of the original trauma, but we may be able to become more responsive each time we are disturbed.

Radical Rest is not a "cure" for trauma, just as it is not a cure for any of the Calls to Rest in this book. It cannot be a cure in part because the philosophy behind Radical Rest is based on an understanding that a human being is such a complex and wonderful creation that there could not possibly be a single "cure." Radical Rest also takes the viewpoint that a human being cannot be measured by the sum of his or her parts. Sometimes parts may feel broken, but in Radical Rest we can begin to believe and feel that our truest self is always whole. We regain some control over how we move our body, we increase our awareness of how we feel within our body, and we can even change the stories we tell about ourselves and our ideas of who we are. We connect deeply with ourselves and realise that the experience of being ourselves is one which is always changing. We are not as fixed as we may believe, and change is always possible. After all, the sun always shines, even behind the clouds.

While some of us may be familiar with feeling broken, ashamed, or worthless, Radical Rest proposes that beneath that feeling of having come apart is a feeling of wholeness and completeness that cannot be taken away once we have connected with it deeply. This wholeness comes from our essence, our soul, the part of us that is immeasurable and cannot be quantified by science. (That said, in 1907 there was a study undertaken, since then known as the 21 grams study, which showed that when the human body dies, it becomes lighter—21g in fact. According to Wikipedia,[4] the study was widely regarded as flawed and unscientific, yet the idea that the soul has a physical weight has gone to become somewhat of an urban legend.)

I think of the part of us which is always whole as the soul. The soul offers us a deep connection of what some call God, others call Spirit, and about a hundred other names in-between. In some philosophical systems the idea of the soul is very much linked with the idea of the mind, yet in the Vedanta school of Hinduism the soul is the true self beyond the ideas created by the mind, and we access the soul when we learn to surrender the efforts of the ego. Yoga is a practical system devised to help us differentiate between ego and soul (known as Ātman in Sanskrit).

When we think and act for others, not just ourselves, when we witness terrible destruction or experience what seems like an insurmountable challenge, yet still find it in ourselves to believe in hope and love, we are identifying with something beyond the ego. It is the part of us that is able to get out of bed every morning and face another day, and the part of us which is fed by faith, hope, and love. Being in nature, connecting in a loving and meaningful way with our fellow humans, giving your loving care to a pet or a plant, taking time to be with yourself—all of these fall into the principles of Radical Rest, and all of these are food for the soul, nourishment for the heart, and can begin to help us back to this beautiful world, to participate, and to love.

Radical Rest

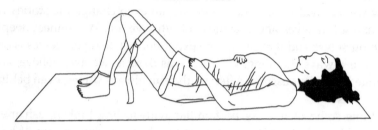

Restorative Yoga posture: Effortless rest.

What you need:

This is one of the simplest postures to try. At most you need a mat to lie on, a support for the head, a strap for the legs and two blocks to support the wrists, but you can really do it without most of those things, providing you can relax without them.

How to do it:

Lie flat on your back, with your legs bent, feet parallel and apart at a comfortable distance away from your bum. Place a neatly folded blanket under your head to support the neck. You may like to support the backs of your hands, just at the crease of the wrist, on two blocks, and tie a yoga strap around the thighs, roughly halfway between hips and knees.

Why it works:

Sometimes the simple things in life are the more rewarding. This posture helps to relieve discomfort in the lower back, and to soften the psoas muscle. When the breath has been caught up in an unhelpful breathing pattern, such as reverse breathing (when the belly rises on the exhale rather than the inhale) or holding the breath, this posture can be a nice way to relax the belly and restore the breath, without you having to think or control the breath in any way.

Watch out for:

Not recommended for women who are heavily pregnant, in the third trimester, or find it uncomfortable to lie flat on their back. If this applies to you, then turn to page 138 and try the posture given for menstrual health.

Also try:

Psoas release on chair (page 57), child's posture (page 68), or the receiving posture (page 138). This is all about feeling safe, so explore with the postures and see what helps you feel the most relaxed. Sometimes a simple savasana as discussed in the section of preparatory postures (page 40) can be a good place to start.

Trauma breathing practice: breath awareness

How to do it:

Start by noticing your breath in its current state. Assess if it is faster, slow, steady, erratic. You may ask, am I breathing through my nose or mouth? Is the breath relaxed or tense? Is my belly moving with my breath? This isn't about getting the right answer, but noticing what is happening in the body at that moment. This practice can be done in the accompanying restorative yoga posture, or simply lying or sitting comfortably. Unlike the other breathing practices given in this book, this practice is a way to begin to become aware of the breath. We do not try to change the breath in any way, rather we just start to notice the breath in its own natural rhythm. You may like to sit quietly for a few moments after, or if you feel tired, lie down and rest.

Why it works:

The more we practise this technique, the more we notice the breath changing throughout the day. We may notice how our belly tenses up if we are in a stressful situation, such as a meeting at work. We may notice how we have been holding our breath as we sit at our computer for a long time concentrating. This awareness helps us over time to realise that we can do small things to adjust and change the breath—such as taking a sigh or a yawn when we notice we have held the breath. This helps to bring us into the present moment, which can bring a great feeling of calm. It also helps us reconnect to our bodies, when we may have disconnected as part of our survival response to a traumatic event.

Watch out for:

With all breathing practices, stop immediately if you feel stressed, anxious, or unwell. Most of us have spent our whole lives not thinking about our breath. To try to force the breath in any way is unproductive. Instead think of this as an invitation to change the flow and direction of the breath. Be curious, and explore what happens. This practice in particular does not have an aim or a goal—it is simply an observation of what is present, in this moment. Be aware that when we bring our mind to the breath, the breath will change slightly. Allow for this to happen, but don't feel you have to adjust the breath in any other way.

Also try:

Once you get comfortable with this practice, you may like to explore some of the others mentioned in this book. Much as with the breathing practices, what works for you may be different from what suits another, so explore, take your time, and remember, you can't get it wrong. If you don't enjoy any of the breath work, just stop. You can always try again another day, or simply try another practice when you feel ready and able. Other breathing practices you might like to try include the exercise given on page 107 in the chapter on grief, or the practice given on page 70 in the chapter on anxiety.

Yoga nidra for trauma:

Please note that going into a trance state may not be helpful for someone who is already really good at dissociating—if you are experiencing a diagnosed form of trauma or working with a therapist of any kind PLEASE seek guidance before starting yoga nidra. Once you are satisfied that this practice may be suitable, please feel free to enjoy it. It is a gentle introduction to yoga nidra, with an emphasis on feeling the body, and practising opening and shutting the eyes while lying down. Access this recording for free via my website www.melskinneryoga.com/free-yoga-nidra and use the password RestIsRadical!

CHAPTER TWELVE

Call to rest: Menstrual health

On a women-only retreat I attended a few years ago, there was a moment when dancing around with other women to blissful music with the Wiltshire countryside laid out in front of us, fluffy sheepskin rugs and yoga props everywhere, I looked around and saw all the beauty there. All shapes, all sizes, all colours, and all ages—these women were relaxed, ecstatic, in full celebration, and it showed in a haze of colour, energy, and movement. It was glorious. And it was rare. I had just turned thirty-three at the time, and it was the first time I had seen anything like it.

Imagine how this world would be if women felt this good about themselves more of the time. If the little girl thinking she's a princess grew up knowing she was as worthy now as she felt back then in her Cinderella dress. Imagine how we could flourish in the right conditions, understanding our hormones and bodies and embracing our monthly cycles, rather than rejecting them. And imagine if this really could make a difference on the Earth, on the soil and the land. Imagine a world not being brutally and greedily exploited for the last dollar. Imagine all of this. And if it all feels like too much, simply imagine how life could be if you understood your own menstrual cycle a bit more, if you knew—really knew—about the contraception you were using, and if any of this information could change your life. I bet the answer is yes.

Let's look at how we can prevent unnecessary suffering for those with a menstrual cycle, and those who live and work with them. For any fellas reading this book, don't be tempted to skip this chapter (and possibly the rest of the book) just because we've started talking about blood and periods. If you're a man and you don't have a menstrual cycle, or a women who, for whatever reason, doesn't have a menstrual cycle, then this still matters to you, because you are likely to spend a fair amount of time with women who are menstruating. And really this is about more than menstruation: our denial of this process, our limiting beliefs of menstruation as merely a "biological function" or worse, a "curse" to be medicated, merely represent how we view women's bodies: as something to be controlled, tamed, and managed.

One of the blessings of my work is to work with women. Time and time again women show up to my workshops or retreats or classes, and I am taught another lesson about vulnerability. I say another lesson when really it's the same lesson over and over again: do not judge. Just because someone's wearing nice leggings or has a fantastic bum it does not mean she has her life together. My women's yoga sessions involve sitting in a circle and sharing how we're feeling that day. Some women talk about the day of their cycle, some women refer to the moon, and some women simply describe their mood or their activities. There have been tears shed at the simple act of sharing, and I am amazed time and time again at the power that comes from simply bringing a group of women together in a safe and nurturing space. One of the prerequisites of the sharing circle is respect, and we always greet and welcome and thank each woman for sharing.

By honouring each woman in the circle, we give each other permission to be vulnerable. To not have to smile and be pretty and presentable and pleasant, but to actually be able to cry, say we feel like crap, that our period is agony, that our job is killing us, that we're exhausted, that we've had a miscarriage, that our pregnancy is nauseating and terrifying; whatever it is that needs to be shared, we share it and we honour it. It might not sound like much, but to be heard, to be seen, and to be acknowledged is one of the greatest gifts we can give each other. When we allow ourselves to compete, to compare, to criticise, and to judge, we are not only damaging ourselves but we are feeding right into the hands of the multinational companies that profit from the one-size-fits-all idea of beauty. By rejecting ourselves and believing that the only way to be successful or attractive is to look like a size eight, big-haired, pouty-lipped, and glassy-eyed version of a woman we are shown on billboards, we are rejecting the beauty that is present in all of us right now.

An important aspect to the way I teach yoga is to educate women about the menstrual cycle, and create a space for women to come together, listen, share, and connect with each other as well as the cycle that lies within themselves. Through this process I have witnessed great vulnerability and great resistance, raucous laughter and tears, and above all a deep desire to know more, learn more, and feel more. There is also anger, for the wisdom that has been taken away from us, the wisdom we were not told at the time of menarche, the first bleed, because our mothers, aunts, sisters, and grandmothers also did not know.

Just another hysterical woman

Blood. Bleeding. Red. Cramps. PMT. PMS. Fertility. Contraception. Hot flushes. Mood swings. How you think and feel about all this stuff, whether you are male or female or non-gender-specific, matters. How we use language matters, and while we're on the topic of language, I'd like to say something about gender.

When I speak of menstrual health in this book, I will use the words women and woman, female and feminine. I am aware that not everyone who bleeds identifies as a woman and that the words female and male, feminine and masculine, have been used to categorise and label in a way that beautiful, complex, and individual human beings cannot be categorised or labelled. Although I do not wish to isolate anyone who does not identify as a woman yet may still bleed, I choose to widely use the words woman and women. This is because I believe these are not negative or denigrating words and I hope that even if you personally do not identify with those words but have a menstrual cycle, the essence of this chapter will still be helpful. In the same way that I have offered people to replace my use of the word soul with psyche, replace any of the words I use with something you feel more appropriate to you.

Most of us don't experience menstruation or menopause as an initiation or celebration. Menstruation has become a curse, an inconvenience, a medical problem to be suppressed and ignored. Despite being one of the reasons our human race survives, menstruation is still a taboo subject, probably only beaten by menopause in its complete and utter banishment from the public arena. We hide tampons up our sleeves and we talk about "down there" in hushed tones and in doing so we conspire to reject and deny our cyclical nature.

We are cyclical beings in more ways than just the menstrual cycle, but certainly the menstrual cycle is one of the most embodied ways we experience this. The monthly flow of blood is a reminder—no matter how hard we try to ignore it with tampons, suppress it with artificial contraception, or push it away with painkillers—of an animal part of ourselves, an ancient and earthy part of ourselves. When we dismiss the experiences a woman has in her body, we dismiss the wisdom of the body. We disparage the real emotional, physical, and mental impact that changes in hormones may be having on that woman's life, and we make her feel small, which is convenient, because when we feel small we often feel powerless, and being powerless makes it easier to manipulate and control us. Advertisers have known this for a long time.

If you are convinced that menstruation is a problem to your productivity, ambition, or even your day to day functioning, and you experience pain, tiredness, tension, and the whole range of other "symptoms" that get classified under the vague title of PMS, premenstrual syndrome, then the idea of simply getting rid of the problem seems very seductive. If we believe menstruation holds us back, we become more receptive to the idea of implanting something in our bodies without fully understanding the risks and side effects, much like many of us take the pill in the same way, with no questioning. I know, because I was on the pill for probably about five years without ever wondering about what this daily injection of hormones was doing to my body and health.

Equally, if we ignore our urge to eat, drink, or go to the toilet because we are so glued to our laptop, if we believe we can work harder and do more if we just push ourselves further, fuelled by caffeine and sugar, then it seems possible that we can survive without sleep, without rest. But as many of us know, there is usually a time limit to how far and how hard we can push ourselves, before our bodies simply say "no more." In the same way, I believe that there is only so long we can suppress and manipulate the natural rhythms of the body before the body starts to protest, through PMT or severe menopausal symptoms.

I have lost count of the number of women who have told me they haven't had a period for a whole year, or sometimes even three whole years. They're not using any contraceptive that would have interrupted the menstrual flow, and they have not been diagnosed with polycystic ovary syndrome (PCOS) or endometriosis or been given any other medical reason: their periods have simply stopped. When they tell me they aren't bleeding and they don't worry about it, I can see the worry and strain in their faces, breaking through the perfectly crafted mask of pretending it doesn't matter. We might believe that our jobs and lifestyles would be easier if we didn't bleed, yet many of us (not all, I know, but many) would pick a regular bleed, even with pain or discomfort, than not, because we know that lack of bleeding is not only cause for biological concern but that without the bleed we are missing the opportunity to release and let go each month, not just of the lining of the womb but also the emotional baggage we have collected that month.

When understood correctly the menstrual cycle can not only become a physical clearing out of the womb but a rebirth of our whole being at a deep soul level. Yep, Tampax haven't told you that have they? Many tribal cultures from the Kogi Indians of Colombia to the Dagara of Burkina Faso honoured the time as a call for women to rest up, and commune with spirit, with a greater wisdom beyond the material world. There is a lot of healing to be done over the ignorance that has been passed to us as information, and the wisdom that has been almost lost. The fact is that many of us have no choice but to start to think differently about this. Endometriosis is one menstrual health illness at an all-time high. According to Endometriosis UK, one in ten women in the UK have the condition, but it takes on average seven and a half years to get a diagnosis, meaning that the women who are suffering spend years dealing with chronic pain, fatigue, depression, and compromised fertility, to name just a few of the symptoms.

These statistics alone show our society's complete disregard for women's bodies. Crippling, debilitating pain once a month for ten per cent of women worldwide (that's 176 million women!) just does not appear to constitute a medical emergency in the system we live within. The products that we are sold to "help" us with our bleed are ironically attributed to women's health problems such as vaginal dryness, vaginal cuts, and the potentially fatal toxic shock syndrome (all of which can be caused by tampons). Many brands of tampons and sanitary towels contain dioxins, which according to the World Health Organization are highly toxic and can cause reproductive and developmental problems, damage the immune system, interfere with hormones, and are also carcinogenic. Not only this, but many sanitary products are bleached white, and non-organic cotton products may come from cotton crops which have been sprayed with pesticides. If you choose your beauty products carefully and go organic in the fruit and veg store, then it makes sense to consider what products you are putting next to or inside your vagina. After all, your skin is the most permeable tissue in your body.

On the physical level, we are often embarrassed about how little we know. Not really knowing where the cervix is, let alone knowing that the cervix moves throughout the month (yep, it genuinely does), not knowing that the pains we may feel mid-cycle are ovulation pains, not realising that the womb and uterus are different words for the same thing. There is so much that was either not taught to us at all or was taught to us in a really embarrassing let's-get-this-over-and-done-with-then way by the teacher who drew the short straw in the staff room—so much that we've simply forgotten or were too embarrassed to ever learn. Either way we have generations of women who simply do not know how their own bodies work, and who get frustrated that the lovers in their lives don't know either. How can we know so much about the difference between a latte and a flat white and so little about our bodies? Could it be our rejection of the female form as somehow shameful, dirty, or dangerous? Using scantily clad women to sell everything from yoghurt to fizzy drinks is not a sign of equality and tampons are not a progressive step forward for women's rights. Until we connect within, be comfortable in our bodies just as they are, we remain caught up in a web of self-loathing and denial.

It may be women who menstruate, and therefore women who have to deal with menstrual disease including endometriosis, polycystic ovaries, absent or irregular periods, painful periods, difficulties in conceiving, and menopausal difficulties (not to mention lack of sexual desire, pleasure, or joy), but when women suffer, we all suffer. Men suffer because their girlfriends, wives, daughters, sisters, mothers, co-workers, and friends are suffering. We all lose out on the possibility of connection that can be brought to us by heartfelt sexual union, open and honest conversation, and understanding and compassion. Men also suffer, because if it's difficult for women to express and embody their femininity, then boy is it tough for men to even admit they have a "feminine side" (let alone learn how to embrace, nurture, and nourish it). When our men and boys aren't allowed to be expressive, emotive, loving, or vulnerable, then we all suffer. It seems as though no one is winning apart from the drug companies and advertising agencies.

If you menstruate and are suffering with any of the issues listed at the beginning of this chapter, you are being called to listen up. If you are male and you live or work or play with any women who are suffering with the list of menstrual problems, you are being called to support them. If you're male or female or define yourself as something else, and you're rejecting your cycles, then pick up the phone y'all, because you are being called.

Premenstrual strength

One of the easiest, simplest, and most effective things for menstrual cycle pain and suffering is to rest more, particularly in the days before and during the actual bleed time. In our desire to be successful, to care for our families, and to live well, we are pushing ourselves to our very limits. You may hate me for saying this, but there's a lot to be gained from befriending your PMS. It is calling us to pay attention, and has even been described by menstrual educator and writer Lara Owens as premenstrual strength! Anger, irritation, and pain are all ways of waking us up. Although it can be tempting to try to ignore and push away uncomfortable emotions, it can ultimately be more beneficial to try actually to feel and stay present with them, although I understand that if you're trying to hold down your job and your family then it may feel almost impossible to go to those places. But if you are experiencing intense and frequent pain then you may have to find a way to create time and space. Ask for help and definitely don't feel like you have to do it alone. Recognising your menstrual cycle as more than just a biological function is a radical act of its own, but if your feelings extend to severe depression, body dysmorphia, suicidal thoughts, or anything else which feels beyond the scope of being manageable, please seek support.

The ecosystem of ourselves

Climate change activists often talk about the need to radically change the way we consume. We have become disconnected from the seasons of the Earth, from the intricate and often delicate ecosystems which sustain our life. I add to this that we have also become disconnected from our bodies, the "Earth" of our own being. No longer able to respond to our ever-changing needs to rest, be that as the sun sets earlier each evening in that descent towards winter solstice, the darkening of the moon each month, or for women the onset of menstruation, we lose our identity and understanding of the unique ecosystem of our body. This loss is tragic not only for ourselves but for humankind as a whole. When we dismiss the experiences we have in our body, we dismiss the wisdom in the body. When we shame ourselves for feeling tired, hungry, or bleeding we disparage the hormonal shifts that may be occurring which make us need more sleep or food or rest. We get confused about what we really need, and we become more susceptible to advertising and consumerism. We may scream until we are blue in the face about the sustainability of the Earth, but what about the sustainability of our bodies?

Rejection of menstruation is a rejection of cyclical health, and belittling of rest is a battle with our circadian rhythms, the biological twenty-four hour rhythm that all living creatures on Earth are reported to have. These are rhythms which affect our behaviour, our performance, our emotions, and our mood, and although we may all operate within a twenty-four hour cycle, our peaks and troughs within that cycle vary from individual to individual. This is why getting to know your body and becoming more aware of your energetic times and your drowsy times is invaluable information that can help you become happier and healthier.

The more we push past our desires to rest, the more we consume. Not just more throwaway coffee cups and convenience food in non-recyclable plastic wrappings but disposable plastic sanitary products. Menstrual products are part of a much bigger plastic problem, as we all know from the heartbreaking images we see of seabirds, turtles, and whales wrapped within unnervingly familiar plastic debris.

Our convenience lifestyle is no longer so convenient. We are, despite how many products Apple can sell us and how fast our Wi-Fi can get, still dependent on this Earth to sustain us, and when we dishonour the great power of the Earth to support us we are essentially abusing that which keeps us here. These problems can seem catastrophic and overwhelming. Our media tend to focus on the news stories with the biggest fear factor, and climate change fits the bill, so when media finally do decide to report on the environmental issues which have been developing for decades it is often with an "It's all doomed" angle. There are many people making positive contributions to the technological and scientific solutions which may help us clean up the oceans and skies, there are more companies striving to make more sustainable food packaging, and there are more and more people of all ages, all genders, all classes, demanding that governments take action. Doing less, needing less, resting more—could this help regain a sense of balance over our hormones as well as supporting the survival of our beautiful planet?

Even if you're not sold on the relevance of the menstrual cycle in today's busy world, or convinced of the politics behind "menstruality," none of us can ignore the environmental impact. Consider these facts from the Women's Network at the Environment Agency:

- Every woman uses, on average, over 11,000 disposable menstrual products, which end up in landfill, or rivers or oceans
- Tampons, pads, and panty liners generate more than 200,000 tonnes of waste per year, and they all contain plastic—pads are around 90 per cent plastic
- In 2010, a UK beach clean-up found an average of twenty-three sanitary pads and nine tampon applicators per kilometre of British coastline.

My contribution to this is to invite you to start to take notice of your own personal environment, of the landscape of your body, and your own cycles. Our Earth may need us to take action—but so do our bodies, mind, hearts, and souls. When we let ourselves use the rhythm of our cycles to guide and support our lives, we open up to the possibility of being able to nourish ourselves both at a psychological and physiological level. We take better care of our bodies, we recognise the link between our sleep patterns and our food cravings, our hormone fluctuations and our digestion. We increase our inner knowing, our capacity to be guided from within, not from the myriad of opinions and experts without, and we become truly holistic.

When we increase our understanding of our needs, realising that our appetites, sex drive, and energy levels change throughout our cycle, we become more conscious in decision making. It becomes easier to know when to start the health kick and when to surrender to an extra hour in bed, when to have salad and when to enjoy cake, when to make love (in a heterosexual relationship) for conception, and when to avoid this time if conception is not of relevance to you. This is called menstrual cycle awareness and can benefit those who menstruate, and those who live or work with those who menstruate.

When I first opened my eyes to menstrual cycle awareness, it was at a workshop with Alexandra Pope, modern day pioneer of menstrual cycle awareness. I had never been to anything like that before, never sat in a circle with women talking so openly about moon cups and blood. I didn't know what "day" of the cycle I was on, I had never heard of the idea that the cycle could be divided into four seasons, winter, spring, summer, and autumn, and I certainly didn't know which was my favourite season and which wasn't. This was the start of a massive shift in my thinking, and alongside nutrition, yoga, rest, and a complete overhaul in the way I live my daily life, I also woke up to the profound power of taking time and space to simply just let my body bleed for a few days each month. I gave up using synthetic tampons and sanitary towels, discovered the wonderful world of moon cups and cloth pads, and reconnected with my blood in a way I had been avoiding for years with contraceptive drugs and tampons, really seeing it, observing its changes in colour, texture, and flow.

This awareness of the changes my body was going through each month awoke an awareness of my changing needs to rest. This awareness for rest coincided with my acceptance of my need to practise a gentler and meditative form of yoga, despite the pressure I felt to be more flexible and strong, like the stereotypical image of a yoga teacher. My period offered me the perfect reason to stop and rest, and helped me to see how little I was resting the rest of the month. However, it wasn't easy to find rest at this time. I sometimes had to make last minute cancellations which was stressful, or found myself becoming upset when I couldn't rest when I "should be" resting. Over time I realised that the world is not as perfect as I want it to be, and that sometimes my bleed would schedule itself at the same time as I was due to teaching a retreat weekend.

Learning how to incorporate rest into my daily life gave me a greater resilience to cope with my period on days when I had to be active and engaging but really wanted to be inward and quiet. Without this awareness, my periods would have become more stressful and inconvenient, and the argument to stop menstruation altogether (very much supported by big drug companies) starts to become more rational and helpful.

Resting all cycle round is pretty essential for most women in our hectic world, but especially at the premenstrual and menstruation phases, when the body is physically more tired and the energy is directed to the soul, where it gathers insights and wisdom. This is a belief that has been held by many cultures, and almost lost in the last 2000 years (the Inquisition, or witch-hunt, can be viewed as the ultimate attempt to destroy women's wisdom and sisterhood). There are so many other courses of action we can take, but if we are exhausted and depleted, change can seem at best overwhelming and at worst impossible. It's why we always start with rest. You may go on to change your mindset about menstruation, change your work patterns, maybe change your whole life, but without coming from a state of consistent and steady energy and without people who support and encourage and love you for doing this brave work, you simply are not going to be able to sustain change of any scale.

How Radical Rest helps

When we give ourselves time and space to "do nothing" we allow for emptiness to open. When we learn the treasures to be found and begin to actively seek out solitude we go against societal expectations. Many women have found that taking time out during menstruation has not only relieved menstrual pain and cramps but has supported the rest of the cycle. Women report experiencing bursts of creativity, of quiet relaxation, and have found it easier to make decisions about relationships, careers, and family that felt difficult before. Deep, nourishing, nurturing rest helps us to return to our bodies. By beginning to rest our bodies, we begin to fully realise what it means to rest, in a deep nourishing way, and it is only by living this experience that we truly are able to see how much we are all in need of it.

Experiencing deep rest can reset our cycle and teach us the power of our wild, raw, and creative side. That part of us has been suppressed for too long. For women to really step into their power, to thrive in the world of business and success, we have to work in a way that respects *us*. The more we chip away at ourselves in order to fit into the world, the more we lose the very essence of our being, that is, the very "us-ness" of us, the source of our true creativity and power and ability to thrive. Anything else is a watered-down version of how great we could be, and if that wasn't enough of a reason for change, then listen

up: our planet is calling. Stop the endless buying of toxic sanitary products, plastic tampon applicators, and painkillers, and open up to a new
way of living, guided by the wisdom of your beautiful body and the
cycles of our amazing Earth.

Radical Rest

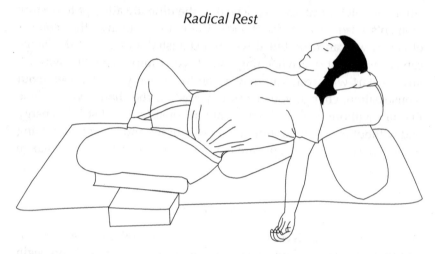

Restorative yoga posture: Receiving posture (in Sanskrit, supported bound
angle pose).

What you need:

This posture works well the more equipment you have, but I find you
can manage perfectly well with lots of cushions and pillows if you don't
have much yoga equipment to play with. If you do have yoga equipment then you need your mat, one or two bolsters, something soft to
support the head (like a thinly folded blanket or light cushion), a strap,
and blocks and bricks to support the thighs. If you don't have that
equipment, that you can manage to do this posture with approximately
three or four firm cushions or pillows, plus something extra to support
the head. When I am really tired in the mornings and can't bring myself
to roll out the yoga mat, I often do this on my bed using pillows.

How to do it:

This posture requires a bit of set-up time, but it really is worth the
effort. Begin by setting up your bolsters or firm cushions into a T-shape

position. These cushions will support your spine and head when you lie back in a few moments, so they must be firm, but with a degree of softness. Sit in front of the T-shaped bolsters and take your knees wide, soles of the feet together. Make sure you have adequate support under the thighs. If you have yoga bricks and blocks these work well, but again, firm cushions also work. If you are using a strap (which is recommended especially if you experience lower back pain), then loop the strap, and pull it over your head to the back of the pelvis. From here, pull it forward and hook it over the little toe side of your feet. Use your arms to gradually take yourself backwards onto the T-shape bolsters— you may need cushions under your arms if your elbows do not touch the floor. Place a folded blanket or thin cushion under the head to support the neck. Pull a blanket over you, take your eye pillow and enjoy. This one's on me. You can stay here for as long as twenty-five to thirty minutes, so long as you have adequate support. The longer you plan to be in the posture the more essential it is that you have plenty of support beneath the legs and arms. Pregnant women can also benefit greatly from this posture, but will need to be extra vigilant and make sure the body is fully supported so there is no overstretching. A nice variation on this posture is to have the legs straight out in front of you, with a bolster under the knees. If you are experiencing any pulling around the pelvis, try this variation instead. When you are ready to come out of the posture, place your hands beneath your thighs and gently lift the knees towards one another. You should be able to step your feet out of the strap. Take your time. When you feel ready, roll carefully to your side and use your arms to push yourself up. Remove the strap and come up to standing nice and slowly.

Why it works:

This posture has seen me through so many exhausted moments. It symbolises our receptivity to nourishment, our willingness to be supported and held. It lengthens the abdomen, opens the chest, and stretches the diaphragm, meaning we can breathe more fully and release any tension or constriction. The opening of the hips allows for a softer inner groin stretch, and encourages the release of menstrual blood as well as the releasing of the lower back. Heavenly for everyone, but especially for women who suffer during their period. I call it "receiving posture," as it really feels like the body is getting a big boost of prana. The traditional name is Supta Baddha Konasana, which means supine bound angle pose, which while descriptive lacks an element of poetry.

Watch out for:

If there are disc problems, avoid having too much lift under the lower back. At menstruation (and in pregnancy) the joints are looser, so having enough support under legs is essential for supporting the pelvis; there should be no sense of pulling in the inner thighs. If you are new to yoga, or have knee injuries, don't stay here for too long, ten to twenty minutes is enough for most people, but if you feel any pulling or pain in your knees, come out of the posture immediately. It can take the knees time to adapt to yoga postures.

Also try:

This posture will open the front of the body, stretching the uterus which can assist with blood flow. For some, it is too open, and they prefer a child's pose (page 68) during their bleed time. As always, explore what works for your body on this particular day. Avoid postures which elevate the pelvis above the heart such as legs-up-wall and bridge-on-chair. If you feel like the downward twist would be of help, then make sure you don't over twist, and keep your belly nice and soft.

Menstrual health breathing practice: flowing circle of breath

How to do it:

Start by noticing your breath in its current state. Judge if it is faster, slow, steady, erratic. You can do this anywhere at any time, including just before you go to sleep. It can even work when you're lying in the bath, or sitting on the bus. Just start to watch each breath, from the start of the inhale all the way through to the end of the exhale, just as if you were riding the big wheel at the fair or stirring your spoon around a big cup of hot chocolate. Inhaling to the top, exhaling to the bottom. Try to stay focused on the whole breath, including the moments you naturally pause and hold the breath. Don't try to hold the breath: you are paying attention to the spontaneous flow of breath, rather than trying to control the breath. You can practise this for at least two minutes up until ten—just make sure you are enjoying the practice and that there is no stress in the breath. You may like to sit quietly for a few moments after, or if you feel tired, lie down and rest.

Why it works:

This breathing exercise can help us focus the mind. By focusing on both inhale and exhale we may notice that the breath naturally becomes longer and slower, but do not try to force this. We can also see the symbolism in the cycle of breath as relating to the menstrual cycle. The inhale is much like the first half of the cycle, a build-up to the peak of the inhale (much like a build-up of energy prior to ovulation), then a letting go of the breath on the exhale, much like the need to let go of the emphasis on material worries and concerns in the second half of the cycle, from ovulation to menstruation.

Watch out for:

With all breathing practices, stop immediately if you feel stressed, anxious, or unwell. Most of us have spent our whole lives not thinking about our breath. To try to force the breath in any way is unproductive. Instead think of this as an invitation to change the flow and direction of the breath. Be curious, and explore what happens.

Also try:

If you are experiencing PMT, then the golden thread breath is marvellous for releasing tension and soothing the mind. It also is a useful birthing breath. Full details of this practice can be found in the book *Yoni Shakti*, but a simple outline is provided here:

- Inhale through the nose, and as you exhale through the mouth, have a slight parting in the lips, and imagine exhaling out a thin golden thread, far out into the space in front of you
- This golden thread can represent any tension, frustration, or anger that you want to express and let go of.

Yoga nidra for menstrual health:

This recording offers the sweet imagery of placing rose petals around the whole of the body as a way of bringing more feelings of nourishment and care towards the being. Access this recording for free via my website www.melskinneryoga.com/free-yoga-nidra and use the password RestIsRadical!

CHAPTER THIRTEEN

Radical Restivism

It could be easy to feel full of despair and gloom at this stage.
After all, we have all known at least one person who has suffered
with a Call to Rest or more, and perhaps we have experienced these
symptoms of restlessness and exhaustion ourselves. We may feel there
is no hope, that the problems we face are too big and unsurpassable,
why bother? We may think that there is a formula to life, and that by
stepping away from the emphasis on doing and achieving we will
somehow lose out, get behind. I say no. There are issues to be tackled
and changes to be made, and there is always, always a step to a brighter
future we can take. Our most powerful moments are in the here and
now. In the words of late poet, Mary Oliver, "Tell me, what is it you plan
to do with your one wild and precious life?"[1]

If you are reading this in the UK, Europe, America, Australia, or
New Zealand, I will make the hopeful assumption you have a roof over
your head and food on your plate. Our politics may not be perfect, but
we still have rights, including the right to vote. We live in a time when it
is far more common to talk about the mind-body connection, the physical world and the energetic world, and the evolution of consciousness.
I use the word common deliberately, as these discussions may have
been going on for thousands of years (yoga is about 5000 years old),[2]

yet it is my understanding that these teachings are no longer limited to the higher castes, the chosen few, but have become the basis for conversations in which we can all begin to discuss and communicate with one another.

There is then hope and light at the end of the tunnel. Yes, perhaps we became disconnected with our bodies and ignorant towards our souls, perhaps our societal values steered us more towards pride, and possession and ownership became our symbols of success over our human qualities of empathy and compassion. Perhaps we became reliant upon doctors to give us the right pills because the drugs seemed so miraculous at the time, and we forgot what it was to heal ourselves with food, herbs, and restoration. Perhaps we gave up on politicians and our belief we could change the world, and became apathetic and despondent—perhaps, perhaps, perhaps, but fear not dear ones because there is always hope within our hearts.

It is hope that keeps us going even in the darkest days. It is hope that lights the candle in our hearts, and it is with hope that we create our day and our life, rather than become a passive bystander. Each day we stand up against the relentless crusade of economics and growth and instead look for the compassion, courage, and creativity that surely encompasses us; we create an inner strength and optimism that cannot be taken away by anything external. Hope comes when we open our hearts and see ourselves more clearly, recognising and accepting ourselves wholly whilst undertaking any healing that we need. Hope arrives when we realise just how beautiful and perfect this planet is for us, and how much we have been given, including fresh air, clean water, and food from the soil beneath us. Hope comes when we can slow down enough in order to wake up and reclaim our right to rest, and in doing so improve our physical, mental, emotional, and spiritual health and find greater ease, satisfaction, and compassion in our lives.

The world thrives on our hopes and our beliefs that things can get better. The abolishment of slavery, the continuing fight for equal rights, the urgency with which the environmental movement is increasing: you don't have to look far to see people all around us hoping to change the world. My personal hope is that this book goes a little way towards offering another look at activism, an activism which recognises that our own health and happiness are critical to the health and happiness of the planet. An activism which requires courage to rest, to slow down, to pause, an activism which doesn't require endless Facebook likes and online click petitions (although they can all be good tools), but rather requires a heartfelt conviction in doing what's right for you, in the belief that you are a precious soul who is more than worthy of being here and that by taking good care of your soul you are already beginning to care for this planet.

I call this type of activism Radical Restivism, a new form of activism that doesn't involve your stress levels going through the roof as you try to take on the world's problems alone. The nine principles of Radical Rest create the moral and philosophical aspirations (as surely all morals and philosophical ideals can surely only ever be aspired towards?), and restorative yoga, breath work, and yoga nidra create the practical and physical application. We have a sense of foundation in the principles, a sense of embodiment in the practices, and the heart and soul in the hope, courage, and love so needed, now as at any time in human history. Such simple and honest words, and yet words that may seem naive, sentimental, and even weak in the times we live in. That may be but sometimes in the midst of world chaos or personal mayhem, hope may be the only thing we can aim for, because even if it feels indulgent, self-centred, or just plain impossible, it is a radical response to the situation we are in and the constant fear we are being sold.

Love has to be recognised as the transformative and uplifting power that it is, and courage has to be dug up from that well deep inside us all—this is about slowing down to wake up, and waking up into a new stream of consciousness that is needed to stop us from sleepwalking our way to personal and environmental chaos, and to find the energy and optimism to *believe* transformation is possible. As Raymond Williams, recognised as one of the most influential thinkers of the New Left, once said, "To be truly radical is to make hope possible, rather than despair convincing,"[3] and in an age of misinformation, "fake news," corruption, and greed, this statement rings true in my ears.

Could doing less really be the key to doing more? I think it's worth a shot. Bringing down our stress levels will be the best preventative medicine we can take for our individual health, and when we are rested the actions we need to take will start to emerge, appearing to us rather like dreams and gifts instead of being desperately pulled from a stressed and frazzled mind. Rather than making decisions from a reactive, tired but wired, and strung-out place, we start to see with greater clarity what exactly we need to do, moment to moment. It is always this moment which helps generate the greatest power (even if you're still lying in bed in your dressing gown).

Beyond the striving and straining and the need to prove ourselves worthy, there is a part of us which is always at peace with who we are right now. Radical Rest takes us there, and the more we can connect with this place, the more we are able to find beauty and contentment in each day, despite the scaremongering in the media and politics in the office. The more we practise Radical Rest the more we are able to see the beauty which surrounds us and the more we realise how much we are a part of that beauty, not separate from nature, but part of nature itself; we are as essential here on the Earth as every tree, plant, and creature.

The more we recognise ourselves as souls, as containing a spark of the Divine, Spirit, God, Universe (or any other word you choose to use), the more we start to live in a way that benefits everyone and everything around us. Slowing down could mean we use less energy, spend less money, buy less, throw away less, drive less, breathe more. Slowing down could see us looking up at the sky, touchiing our hands to the earth beneath our feet, and connecting to our hearts, our hopes, and our dreams. Much like children, we may be able to take pleasure in the simplest of things, to express ourselves clearly and openly, and to love with the whole of our heart. This is Radical Rest, and the power of doing less, to do more.

Remember this: to live each day half-heartedly, to deny your purpose in this life, to reject your creativity, your unique beauty, and your ability to love fully is to slowly deaden yourself. To step forward and live courageously and determinedly, to find the joy and laughter, to embrace the sorrow and grief, to be angry and yet be respectful—this is what will change our lives, and perhaps even change the world. We are in the middle of a system which thrives by controlling us: feeding us negative, limiting beliefs, setting us up to compare and compete, and selling us a fake idea of success, prosperity, and happiness—but this system is collapsing. We see it in our banking systems, in our political systems, and our increasingly unstable environment. It may seem like the world is about to end, but what if it's simply changing, evolving, and rising up from the patriarchal systems and archaic infrastructure that no longer serves us? What if we as human beings are evolving, changing the way we think, move, and act day to day?

If that seems a bit too radical for you right now, then think back to your grandparents' era and how different things were. Chances are your lifestyle is completely different, down to where you live, the work you do, the food you eat, and the way you engage with technology. I grew up with my grandparents, and there is very little in my life today that resembles the way we grew up. We had no car, my Grandad grew most of our fruit and vegetable, we didn't go abroad, we rarely, if ever, ate out (Uncle Ben's curry sauce was considered exotic), and significantly, there were no mobile phones, no social media, and until I was about fourteen, no email. While we could certainly have an interesting conversation about what has been gained and what has been lost, we would probably all agree that life feels faster now, and perhaps we could attribute this back to the changes we saw when we started measuring time, when we slowly, but surely, began to move to the rhythm of the clock rather than the rhythm of the soul.

Whether we are truly busier or not and whether we are in greater crisis now than at other points in our history actually means very little compared to how we perceive life to be right now and if we are tired, stressed and worried, then it's unlikely we can feel full of hope. Until we take the time to reduce our stress levels, find our full and natural breath, and bring steadiness to the mind, we risk clouding our clarity of all the hope and possibility there is available, and risk living a life with the glass half-empty, a life barely felt.

By reducing stress, balancing hormones, and releasing muscular tension, we help ourselves to breathe again. Full deep breathing helps us to bring clarity to the mind, helping us to realise what we can and cannot control within our own lives. We might not single-handedly reduce the amount of plastic in the sea, but there *is* always an action we can take in each moment. We are always making decisions, day in, day out. If we can make those decisions from a relaxed and calm place, with a heart full of love and hope, then couldn't it be possible that our entire life could change right before our eyes? And I don't mean big external life changes necessarily (although that could be the case), but I mean the inner changes, the inner shifts, the move towards greater self acceptance. If we begin to just think what it means to treat our land with respect by learning to respect our bodies, if we act with kindness, without any pressure to be perfect to get things right, if we take time to sit quietly or rest deeply for a few minutes every day: these small actions can and have changed lives. Radical Rest is not only a joyful thing to welcome into your life, but it could be an essential thing to help us prepare for the challenges that lie ahead.

The time for yoga is now

In the *Yoga Sutras*, a philosophical text often taught to yoga teachers-in-training, it states that the time for yoga is now. It is always now and you are never more powerful than you are in this moment. So let's take a moment to feel this moment. Perhaps your belly is full of fire and your heart is beating, maybe the mind feels awake, alert, intrigued, and alive or maybe you are realising just how tired you really are.

Regardless of what we may believe we all have the ability to make a choice in every moment. Without a doubt the subconscious is playing out in our words and actions but we do have a degree of choice available to us. We can elevate our consciousness, increase our awareness, and begin to let ourselves rest. We can observe the effects of our actions and realise that we can choose a different way, forge a different path, start to let go of our pain and suffering, and move through our emotions fully and wholly because we know we are so much more than that which defines us.

So, you've set your intention. You start to rest.

Let's say that against all the odds you've figured out how to carve out a little bit of time to yourself, perhaps starting with a weekly yoga class or making a habit of practising yoga nidra once or twice a week before you go to bed. You've accepted that there may be some pain that rises to the surface, some healing to be done, and you step up to the challenge with the nine principles to support you. Your courage is accompanied by some nervousness and your compassion is not without criticism, because we all know that change can be hard work, and some part of our self remembers that transformation comes with fire and fire sometimes burns. Remember though, fire also purifies.

Days go by, weeks, maybe years. Sometimes it feels like nothing is happening, you wonder what's the point, wouldn't it be better to be keeping up with everyone else, trying to slim down your hips and belly, earn more money, get the kids into a better school, or buy a bigger house. Sometimes you think about going back to your old ways, but you can't quite bring yourself to do it. Some days you feel so full of hope and light and love that you forget how it used to be, to be so weighed down, so hopeless and numb—and then those sensations return to visit you and remind you to stay attentive because every day is a new day and *all* our sensations are simply a part of our human experience.

Respect yourself if you are even considering that idea of incorporating Radical Rest into your life: it requires courage to stand up in the face of the status quo and say, no, I do not want to do that. It requires honesty, as we assess how much of our free time is spent pursuing conscious rest, and how much is spent with activity that depletes us. This is about stepping away from all you've ever been sold that no longer fits and instead finding peace with yourself exactly as you are. In other words we start to accept our flaws, acknowledge our traumas, forgive our bad habits, and stop worrying quite so much about what other people think. The most important acceptance we can find is the acceptance we give ourselves.

Remember this: you are not broken and you do not need fixing. Perhaps you need help with symptoms—your achy back, your chronic fatigue, your trauma, or your anxiety, and so yes, these symptoms do need healing, but you are so much more than your symptoms, you are a soul residing in this world, and souls can never be broken. Recognise that we are all doing the best we can, in this often bizarre, heartbreaking, frustrating human life, and remember that beneath this chaos and confusion, there is a greater peace, like an island of stillness amid stormy seas. Radical Rest can take you there—if you let it.

My journey to Radical Rest was extreme—I gave up a career I had worked tirelessly for, practised Radical Rest at least once a day for over five years (before I even knew what it was), and ended up writing this book. Your journey need not be so extreme, your experience not so radical. For many people, learning how to make rest a regular part of life will make a massive difference to their mental, emotional, and physical health, and this could be enough. You don't need to take on the world—but if you feel so inclined, remember that without community, connection, and consciousness our efforts are often short-lived.

However we choose to practise Radical Rest (and there are more practical tips coming up in the next chapter), we are choosing to wake up to slow down. We are lying down to wake up. And there is so much beauty to wake up to, from the wildness of our Earth to the far off sun, moon, and stars, and to the beauty of connection with one other. Let's open our eyes to how much we have, and how much we could lose, and use Radical Rest to delve into the resting place of the soul, because from this place anything and everything is possible.

When I was in the Aran Islands, on the yoga nidra intensive training which initiated this book, I wrote this poem, and it somehow feels right to end the book on this. Thank you for reading.

To those who dare
To spread their wings
And fly a little higher,

To those who jump
In rivers and streams
And stand gazing at the fire.

To those who scatter stones and sticks
And leave marks where they tread,
To those who aren't afraid to live
And know that they're not dead.

To those whose hearts soar and sing
To those who rest and play
To those that find their work in love
And find joy in every day.

To those who shout and laugh and cry
Who smile hello
And smile goodbye,
To those made of earth, water, fire and air

This is for the ones that dare.

CHAPTER FOURTEEN

Radical Rest toolkit

Now you're all signed up to Radical Restivism, below is a suggestion of some tools to help you begin your journey. Only buy what you feel you need and don't be worried if you can't afford or simply don't want to buy any stuff. I have practised in all sorts of places often with very little, if any, yoga equipment, but it's amazing how cushions and pillows can create bolsters, how scarves act as eye pillows, and couches and futons and even beds make very good alternatives to yoga mats. Be discerning with your shopping choices, and love what you buy.

- **Headphones**
  Some people like to use headphones when listening to yoga nidra. I've never been a fan of having things in my ears, but I have used headphones when using yoga nidra on public transport, including planes, and have even managed to nidra my way through an eight hour plane journey to India before!

- **Eye pillow**
  These are little cushions that rest either directly on the eyes or on the eyebrows to provide shade and weight to soften the front brain,

help the eyes to relax, and take us more quickly to a quiet place. You can buy them online, but often yoga studios sell them, and people sometimes even make them, so ask around. You could even make your own—there's lots of stuff online showing you how.

- **Blanket**
  I buy blankets from a fellow yoga teacher in Bristol for my retreats, and nearly always sell them on during retreats because the students just fall in love with them. Blankets are one of those things that can be expensive or cheap, but there is a huge variety out there, so get stuck in. I tell the students on retreat to associate the blanket with a time of rest and this can really encourage us to settle into the practice of yoga nidra at home more regularly.

- **Journals**
  Journals are a great way to begin to build a relationship with our thoughts and beliefs and a crucial tool for anyone looking to chart their menstrual cycle beyond the multitude of apps available. They are also a great tool for the practising of gratitude and positive affirmations—more on that below.

- **Gratitude and positive affirmations**
  Gratitude is such an important quality to bring into our lives. Start with step one, looking around and seeing all you have been given, from the clothes on your back to the food on your plate. When we start learning how to be grateful for everything we have in our lives right now, we stop needing things to be different before we think we can be happy. It is pretty simple: every day, either in the morning or before you go to bed, write a list of everything you've been grateful for that day. You don't have to come up with brand new things every day—in fact there's something to be said for recognising day in, day out just how much food is available to most of us, the roof over our heads, and so on. The next step will emerge without your effort, and this is gratitude for life itself. Don't force this step—but be open to the idea. You never know, you could one day surprise yourself.
  Positive affirmations are statements of belief, usually in yourself and your ability, and somewhat surprisingly for a culture so focused on the mind, many of us find it easy to be cynical or dismissive about affirmations. There are increasing numbers of neuroscientists and linguists researching this field, and certainly celebrities like

Oprah Winfrey and even Arnold Schwarzenegger are not shy about sharing their habit of using positive affirmations as tools in their success. Personally I love working with positive affirmations as a daily practice because it is so easy for me to slip into "glass half empty" thinking without realising it, and getting stuck there for some time. You can find out more about the power of positive thinking from Louise Hay's book, *You Can Heal Your Life*, which also shares Louise's inspiring personal story.

Certainly as we become more aware of the power of our thoughts in creating our life, it seems as though positive affirmations could be not just useful, but invaluable in helping us change the way we look at the world. This isn't to say you have to deny or ignore any thoughts or emotions that feel "negative," this would certainly not be healthy or helpful, but to balance out the perhaps more familiar and established critical voice with a refreshing and optimistic one. Over time, and with regular practice of the other components of Radical Rest, we can learn to welcome in our whole experience without overly judging or shaming ourselves.

- **Yoga mat**
Some people are devout yogis but just cannot get into the habit of practising at home. I love my home practice, and over the years my yoga mat has become a trusted friend. If you just plan to practise yoga nidra, you technically don't need a yoga mat, but sometimes it can be nice to have a special place that you go to take rest, especially if you plan to get some of the other suggestions on the list, like an eye pillow or bolster. If you are going to buy a mat, they range in price—think about what you're going to be using it for when you buy. If you're going to buy something that is just for lying on, you might not need the most expensive. If you plan to practise hatha yoga (the more physical kind), then something with a bit of grip may be more suitable.

- **Bolster**
Bolsters are at the more expensive end of yoga kit to buy—but they are pretty special. They are basically like big cushions that, in yoga nidra, are great to place under the backs of the knees so that the lower back feels more comfortable. You probably only need one, and it would make a good Christmas or birthday present to ask for. If you have firm cushions and pillows at home, you can make do with those most of the time.

- **Yoga chair**
  This may seem an unnecessary piece of kit, but for the serious restorative yoga devotee, it can become invaluable. Don't feel under pressure to get one—there are many ways to practise Radical Rest which are inexpensive and don't require buying things. I offer alternatives to postures involving a chair throughout the book.

- **Workshops and sessions with me**
  I run regular workshops and retreats and offer one-to-one work. You can find out more about those, and sign up to my monthly newsletter *Moon Mail* which arrives in your inbox every new moon with a free yoga nidra offering, blog, and updates. Sign up via my website. http://www.melskinneryoga.com/

Radical Rest: other ways to practise

There are also other ways to find Radical Rest—the suggestions below are a few of my personal favourites, but I'd love to hear yours. Share your ideas with me via email mel@melskinneryoga.com.

- **Sleep**
  There is nothing better than sleep. Even yoga nidra cannot replace regular, decent sleep. Do not deprive yourself. Do not cast sleep somewhere below watching *Game of Thrones* on your list of priorities. This is true soul food. Make your bedroom peaceful, not too hot or too cold, and wind down for bedtime as though something special is about to happen because it is: the world of dreaming awaits, the place of restoration is calling you, and the healing wants to happen. Don't delay.

- **Napping**
  I once heard yoga nidra referred to as yoga nidra naps. I freely admit that I have on more than one occasion settled down to listen to a recording of yoga nidra, dozed off, and woken halfway through the next recording. As much as I may have the intention to be awake and aware, I love the feeling of knowing I just got some serious rest time. Alternatively you can just set your timer and lie down for a good old-fashioned nap. Choosing the length of your nap is essential to avoid grogginess—for maximum geek factor, read the fascinating

book *Take a Nap, Change Your Life*, which offers you a scientific way to work out the perfect nap time for your needs.

- **Food**
  Mmm food. A troubled area for many I know, but also an opportunity for such self-care. Not only in terms of deciding what to eat, but also finding joy in the act of eating. I know supermarkets may not be much fun, but you can find pleasure in having so much choice, desire in what you choose to eat, honour in cooking each meal, and gratitude in eating. Let it be restful activity, not a chore. The repetition of chopping vegetables is very soothing as is stirring a bowl of soup or risotto. Most of us can't stop our busy lives at the push of a button—but we can find rest in our actions.

- **Music**
  We are all rhythmic creatures, and regardless of your held beliefs about whether you can or cannot sing or dance or play an instrument, I urge you to explore the joys of music. Whether you go to a dance class, make your own drum, or dance around your kitchen in the morning, let music lead you back to the rhythm of your heart. Conscious movement can be as re-energising as Radical Rest when done with heartfelt joy.

- **Nature**
  Find a place with trees, running water, birdsong, and clean air, and keep going back because this is where healing happens. This is the place where my inner poet rejoices and where I wake naturally at sunrise and want to walk for hours. It's where if I am menstruating I can lie on my back on the earth for hours, needing nothing else. It is magical and without it we become hardened and tense. Walk barefoot, watch the sun rise, gaze at the moon, and enjoy watching the trees change shape over the seasons. Soon you will start to realise that you are not in nature but you are nature.

- **Creativity**
  Reading, drawing, painting, cooking, writing, singing, playing music … we can be creative in almost anything that we do. Think back to what you liked doing as a child, and consider starting that hobby up again, for pleasure, not achievement.

- **Mindfulness meditation**
  This can be another fantastic tool. It teaches us how to understand and manage our mind so it becomes our friend rather than our enemy. When we become less caught up in our thoughts, we are better able to respond to situations (not react), to set boundaries (what we do with our time), and also to acknowledge our own power in each moment to make those choices. There are several courses you can take, as well as lots of offerings on platforms like YouTube, Headspace and more.

- **Baths**
  A hot bath filled with Epsom salts and essential oils can be exquisite. If you use Epsom salts, make sure you rehydrate with lots of water and rest afterwards and check the health warnings on the packet. If you don't have a bath, you can use Epsom salts as a foot soak, or alternatively try dropping a few drops of essential oil in the shower before you turn on the water—the scents should fill the room creating a spa-like effect in your own bathroom. Water is incredibly healing, especially for those water signs out there (I'm looking at you Pisces, Cancer, and Scorpios).

- **Rituals and ceremonies**
  For those of you that are shuddering at the idea of dancing naked around the fire, fear not because I don't mean that sort of ceremony (necessarily). We have ceremonies and rituals in everyday life without realising—not just birthdays and Christmas but going to the pub for drinks on Friday night after work, the weekly yoga class, the yearly holiday abroad: all of these things are rituals which feed us in some way. Why not create different types of rituals? New moon and full moon rituals are really popular now, and they are easy to do. Anything goes, and you'll find loads of suggestions online and in some of the books on menstrual health I list at the back, but generally I like to light smudging sage and cleanse my home with it, light some candles, and do some meditation to prepare.
  New moon is thought to be the time of bringing in what you desire, so you could try writing it down or drawing a picture and putting it somewhere safe, and full moon symbolises the time to let go of anything which is getting in the way of that desire—again you could write or draw whatever you feel is blocking you, then burn it

or tear it up. Be specific, and enjoy it! At the end it can be nice to have a dance, a bath, a bit of chocolate … whatever you like, really.

- **Conscious menstrual consumerism**
  If you menstruate then it's worth thinking seriously about your menstrual product consumption. There are great books about this, which I've listed in the radical reading list, but essentially most sanitary items (think towels and tampons) are designed to be thrown away so that you have to keep buying, month after month, year after year, decade after decade. More and more entrepreneurial women out there are creating fun, environmentally friendly products that can be reused. Moon cups and cloth pads are just two ways you can help save the planet (whilst avoiding soaking up all the chemicals that are on most white-as-white sanitary towels and tampons) and protect your bank balance.

- **Eat well**
  With regards to food, we can all make small changes to how we shop, from supporting your local stores, buying organic and/or seasonal, buying only what you need, recycling food waste, avoiding plastic, growing your own … there are no lectures here, just a suggestion that while we're not here to save the world on our own, surely no harm can come from us all trying to do our bit?

- **Sex**
  Yep, good old sex is incredibly restful for the mind and the body. Who'd have thought it? If you don't have a partner, go solo, I dare you.

- **What not to do**
  Sometimes rest is just about what you don't do, such as the use of technology. My phone spends most of its life quite happily on flight mode, until I need it, and then I respond to whatever comes through. It's relatively early days when it comes to truly knowing whether being attached to a mobile phone has a negative impact on the health but I for one enjoy the days I turn my phone off and after a few days of just checking my phone once a day find I become much more calm and relaxed. Find the happy medium that suits your lifestyle, but remember that for many decades phones were something we walked past in our house, not something we were required to look at every five minutes.

Ultimately, don't try to do too much! The list above is simply some ideas of what you might like to do. Radical Rest isn't meant to be another thing on the to-do list that causes stress and anxiety. While you might have to make time for Radical Rest in the beginning, don't try to do too much at once. Remember—doing less is the new doing more.

ACKNOWLEDGEMENTS

I have to start with a big thank you to my husband, Nick for your love and support, kindness, encouragement, and humour. And for our home—our lounge/office/yoga room/art space/dining room (!) has supported us through a lot.

Thank you to Polly for the beautiful illustrations, to Alice Guthrie for your kind and gentle feedback on the book on its very early days, and to Elisabeth Brooke for your very generous guidance, advice and support. To Aeon Books, for making this a real book and not just a Google Doc! To my yoga teachers: Laura Gilmore for helping me take my first steps along this wild and amazing path of yoga, Uma Dinsmore-Tuli for taking me to the Aran Islands to begin with, and James Reeves for the first iRest yoga nidra training.

To every space that has ever held my teachings, especially Bristol City Yoga. I'm lucky I never had to go to India to find my spiritual home! To everyone who has helped make my workshops and retreats so luscious. Gladey for the beautiful blankets, and Milly for the ever popular chocolate truffles, bringing extra amounts of nourishment to my workshops.

To Lynn and Kira, two incredible healers who have helped me deeply, and to my grandparents and my mum, for the foundation of love which continues to carry me on.

All my friends in Brizzle, Kernow and those in distant lands ... I love you. To Poppy, for the sharing of your family! To Tom, Will, Owen, and Sam for accepting me into the tribe and of course to Jane, for absolutely everything (not forgetting Lizzie of course—if it's possible for a dog to be a soulmate, I met mine).

To Rosie Walsh, writer, student, inspiration, for your incredibly clear advice on publishing vs. self-publishing, and for not laughing when I told you I was writing a book.

For the Shropshire Hills, the Tamar Valley, the Cotswolds: being held in the beauty of these landscapes helped me so much. To Hawkwood College, for not only being the home of my first ever retreat, but also for the artists' residency. Thank you so much.

For the teachers I did not meet but who influenced me through their words and practices, including of course the original yogis. And of course, to everyone who has ever come to class, come to a workshop, come on retreat, braved one-to-one work with me, and who offered to help with this book: thank you so much. I love my work, and it's only because of you I get to call this my work.

And finally thanks to *you* for reading this book. You made it to the end. Well done. I'd love to stay in touch. You can email me at mel@melskinneryoga.com or through my website www.melskinneryoga.com.

RESTFUL RADICAL READING

These are some of the books that have helped shine a light on my journey as I stumbled through the dark.

Women's health and menstrual awareness

The Red Tent, Anita Diamant
If Women Rose Rooted, Sharon Blackie
Yoni Shakti, Uma Dinsmore-Tuli
The Optimised Woman, Miranda Gray
Awakening Shakti, Sally Kempton
Code Red, Lisa Lister
Women's Bodies, Women's Wisdom, Christine Northrup
Her Blood Is Gold, Lara Owen
Women Who Run with the Wolves, Clarissa Pinkola Estes
Wild Genie, Alexandra Pope
Wild Power, Alexandra Pope and Sjanie Hugo Wurlitzer
Women, Food and God, Geneen Roth

Creativity

Big Magic, Elizabeth Gilbert

Physical, mental, and spiritual health

A Mind of Your Own, Kelly Brogan
The Brain that Changes Itself, Norman Doidge
Stumbling Stones: a Path through Grief, Love and Loss, Airdre Grant
How to Heal your Life, Louise Hay
The Psoas Book, Liz Koch
Anatomy of the Spirit, Caroline Myss
Why Zebras Don't Get Ulcers, Robert M. Salpolsky
The Mind Body Workbook, Debbie Shapiro
Radical Remission, Kelly A. Turner, PhD
Yoga for Depression, Amy Weintraub

Politics, culture

Happy People, Healthier Planet, Tessa Belton
The Happiness Industry, William Davies
When Society Becomes an Addict, Ann Wilson Schaef

Poetry

Benedictus, John O'Donogue
Everything Is Waiting for You, David White
The Poetry Pharmacy, William Sieghart
Soul Food, edited by Neil Astley and Pamela Robertson-Pearce
Rumi: The Essential Rumi, Coleman Barks

Sleep and rest

The Power of Rest, Matthew Edlund, PhD
The Radical Pursuit of Rest, John Koessler
Take a Nap! Change Your Life, Sara C. Mednick PhD

Trauma

The Body Keeps the Score, Bessel van der Kolk
Waking the Tiger, Peter Levine
The iRest Program for Healing PTSD, Richard C. Miller, PhD

Yoga and spirituality

The Science of Yoga, William J. Broad
Polishing the Mirror, Ram Dass
The Heart of Yoga, T. K. V. Desikachar
The Bhagavad Gita, Eknath Easwaran
The Breathing Book, Donna Farhi
The Sabbath, Abraham Joshua Heschel
Light on Yoga, BKS Iyenger
Eastern Body Western Mind, Anodea Judith
Relax and Renew, Judith Lassiter Hanson
Yoga Nidra, Richard Miller
Hell Bent, Benjamin Lorr
Yoga Sutras, Matthew Remski
Waking, Matthew Sanford
Yoga Body, Mark Singleton
Yoga Nidra, Swami Satyananda Saraswati

NOTES

Chapter One

1. Cited in Tara Brach, *Radical Self-Acceptance* (p. 24).
2. https://instagram.com/explore/tags/wellness/?hl=en
3. https://theguardian.com/lifeandstyle/2017/sep/17/yoga-better-person-lifestyle-exercise

Chapter Two

1. John O'Donohue, *Benedictus* (p. 140). Excerpt from poem, For One who is Exhausted.
2. Elizabeth Gilbert, *Big Magic*.

Chapter Three

1. https://sleepcouncil.org.uk/wp-content/uploads/2018/04/The-Great-British-Bedtime-Report-2017.pdf

Chapter Four

1. Matthew Edlund, *The Power of Rest* (p. 12).

Chapter Five

1. Donna Farhi, *The Breathing Book* (p. 5).

Chapter Six

1. Anodea Judith, *Eastern Body Western Body* (pp. 18–19).
2. *The Yoga Sutras of Patanjali*, translated by Sri Swami Satchidananda (sutra 1.2, p. 4).
3. Attributed to Henry Ford.
4. https://ted.com/talks/kelly_mcgonigal_how_to_make_stress_your_friend Ted talk

Chapter Seven

1. Gabor Mate, *When the Body Says No* (p. 5).

Chapter Eight

1. http://bbc.com/future/story/20160909-why-you-feel-busy-all-the-time-when-youre-actually-not
2. Eknath Easwaran (translated), *The Upanisahds* (p. 57).

Chapter Nine

1. William Davies, *The Happiness Industry* (p. 143).
2. Tias Little, *Yoga of the Subtle Body* (p. 174).

Chapter Ten

1. Robert M. Sapolsky, *Why Zebras Don't Get Ulcers* (p. 221).
2. William Davies, *The Happiness Industry* (p. 178).

Chapter Eleven

1. Bessel van der Kolk, *The Body Keeps the Score.*
2. Peter Levine, *Waking the Tiger, Healing Trauma* (p. 143).
3. For more on this see Norman Doidge, *The Brain that Changes Itself.*
4. https://en.wikipedia.org/wiki/21_grams_experiment

Chapter Thirteen

1. Mary Oliver, *Wild Geese*, cited in *Soul Food* (p. 36).
2. Mark Singleton, *Yoga Body* (p. 25).
3. Raymond Williams, *Resources of Hope* (p. 118).